Praise for **Sustainable Wellness**

"Matt Mumber and Heather Reed have taken the heart of integrative medicine and put it into action by reflecting on their life work and writing this beautiful book together. With inspiring teaching stories, thoughtful questions, and practical exercises they teach us how to get well or stay well."

—Victoria Maizes, MD; executive director, Arizona Center for Integrative Medicine; professor of Clinical Medicine, Family Medicine, and Public Health, University of Arizona

"At long last a manual on the fine details of wellness! Supported by an extensive bibliography and years of experience, the authors lay out a series of tools to help guide those of us in need of refocusing our lives. The language is explicit, succinct, and easily comprehensible by everyone regardless of background. Healthcare professionals will particularly be enthralled with the easy-to-follow suggestions that cover topics in detail not discussed elsewhere. A book for the 21st century and beyond that you will come back to often. I thank the authors for their time and dedication and the readily apparent passion they display throughout this scholarly book. It is truly a must read."

—Alfonso Diaz, MD, FACC, medical director, Harbin Clinic

"*Sustainable Wellness* is a must-read book for all. [Mumber and Reed] have written a captivating book that is easy to read and full of great advice! They clearly describe practical ways we can all improve ourselves and become healthier and happier human beings. They cover in detail the ways to reach sustainable wellness through nutrition, physical activity, and stress management."

—Omer Kucuk, MD; professor of Hematology-Oncology and Urology; leader, Prostate Cancer Research Program; director, Multidisciplinary Genitourinary Oncology Group; chief, Genitourinary Medical Oncology, Winship Cancer Institute, Emory University

"*Sustainable Wellness* offers a refreshingly mature and practical synthesis of wisdom from the field of integrative healthcare. The authors' genuine caring and experience shine through as they illuminate proven pathways to living with greater mindfulness and satisfaction, no matter what current health challenges we may face. In a crowded field, this book stands out as exceptionally reader-friendly and inspiring. I highly recommend it to all who wish to live life to the fullest."

—William Collinge, PhD; author of *Partners in Healing*; founder of the Touch, Caring & Cancer Program

"From the voices of two masterful healers, readers hear the simple truths that enable us to achieve the health and wellness we so desire. Because Matt and Heather clearly serve others and navigate their own journeys of health and healing, their approach is simultaneously practical and profound. What I admire most about their work is that it leaves me with renewed confidence in myself as a healer. It's the most empowering feeling to recognize that 'I am the healer I am seeking' and have the tools and knowledge to make it so!"

—Nancy M. Paris, MS, FACHE; president & CEO, Georgia Center for Oncology Research and Education (Georgia CORE)

"In *Sustainable Wellness*, Dr. Matt Mumber draws on his many years of personal and professional experience to offer a powerful, inspiring approach to creating sustainable body/mind/spirit health and wellbeing. His vision of whole-person medicine is a gift for anyone seeking a healthier, more authentic, and more fulfilling life. Individuals, and medicine as a whole, will benefit greatly from his wisdom, caring, and insights."

—Jeremy Geffen, MD, FACP; medical oncologist; author of *The Journey Through Cancer*

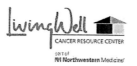

LivingWell
CANCER RESOURCE CENTER
part of
ℝ Northwestern Medicine

"Dr. Matt and Heather Reed understand that achieving and maintaining sustainable wellness requires that we go beyond the current doctor (teacher) and patient (submissive sufferer) paradigm. This wonderful book artfully explains why health starts within oneself; why a patient-centered approach to care is best achieved with true physician collaboration; and how self-efficacy can be practiced and beneficial in myriad ways, based on each person's unique makeup."

—Glenn Sabin, cancer survivor; founder of FON therapeutics

"*Sustainable Wellness* is a breath of fresh air in the healthcare field. Clearly written with simple suggestions, it opens the door to recognizing that wellness is available to each person, right now!"

—Janice L. Marturano, executive director, Institute for Mindful Leadership

"As the spouse of a 10-year cancer survivor and as a collaborator with Dr. Mumber, I have seen his integrative approach to sustainable wellness at work in two different aspects of my life and that of my wife. I'm delighted that he and Heather Reed have written this book, so that you don't need to have cancer or engage in a research project to learn these life tools. I have been surprised and impressed by the power that these tools provide in my life."

—John Grout, The David C. Garrett Professor and Dean of the Campbell School of Business, Berry College

"Dr. Matt and Heather draw on their experiences and practices to provide a well-marked path to health. This book gives readers confidence and inspiration to follow their own journey to wellness. I highly recommend it to all who wish to find that most elusive jewel of life: balance."

—Ken Davis, MD; CEO, Harbin Clinic LLC

"The world has been waiting for this book. It is not just a support and self-care manual for living life in ways that sustain health and well-being; *Sustainable Wellness* guides the reader on an easy, steady, and comfortable journey that makes the going as joyful as any imagined destination."

—Jnani Chapman, RN, BSN; senior staff member of Commonweal; founder and Director of YCat Yoga Therapy Training Program

"*Sustainable Wellness* removed me from my frightening path of cancer. It brought my mind, body, and spirit back to living. I am a lady in my 60s and for the first time in my life I really wrapped my mind around the concept of breath. I finally understand the gift of breath being with me from my moment of birth until my last breath at death. I finally understand the respect my breath is due from me as an individual. Now I can close my eyes, take conscious breaths in and out, and physically and spiritually rejoice at the sounds, feelings, and wellness my breath provides me throughout each day. The program taught me how to cultivate awareness for the remainder of my time. I thank Dr. Matt and Heather for sharing the warmth in their hearts and the knowledge in their minds. They gave me the support that I needed to once again see the light on this beloved Earth and to trust bringing conventional, complementary, and alternative medicine together. I found my smile again!"

—Linda Gray, group and retreat participant

SUSTAINABLE

Wellness

SUSTAINABLE

Wellness

AN INTEGRATIVE APPROACH
to
Transform Your Mind, Body, and Spirit

MATT MUMBER, MD
AND HEATHER REED

Foreword by Dr. Andrew Weil

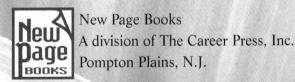

New Page Books
A division of The Career Press, Inc.
Pompton Plains, N.J.

SUSTAINABLE WELLNESS
EDITED AND TYPESET BY KARA KUMPEL
Cover design by Howard Grossman/12E Design
Printed in the U.S.A.

Poem on page 214 excerpted from *The Cup of Our Life* by Joyce Rupp. © 1997 by Ave Maria Press, Inc., PO Box 428, Notre Dame, Indiana, 46556, *www. avemariapress.com*. Used with permission of the publisher. All rights reserved.

Enneagram chart and QUEST test © 2012 by The Enneagram Institute. Used with permission.

To order this title, please call toll-free 1-800-CAREER-1 (NJ and Canada: 201-848-0310) to order using VISA or MasterCard, or for further information on books from Career Press.

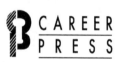

The Career Press, Inc.
220 West Parkway, Unit 12
Pompton Plains, NJ 07444
www.careerpress.com

Library of Congress Cataloging-in-Publication Data

CIP Data Availale Upon Request.

Dedicated to the ground of awareness.

Acknowledgments

Our deepest gratitude goes to our families, in particular Laura Mumber and Len Pojunas, for their unwavering support.

Our appreciation goes to the many retreatants and group participants who continue to humble and inspire us and to the board and staff of Cancer Navigators, especially Denise Powers, for the many ways they support the work.

Our thanks go to Orbert Rogers for his invaluable technical support and to Jim Clewell for his artistry. Thank you to our extended family of volunteers for their gift of time, especially Ethel Evans and LeAnn Yeargan.

We remember our many teachers and mentors, especially Dr. Bernie Siegel, Thich Nhat Hanh, Dr. Rachel Remen, Dr. Andrew Weil, Ken Wilber, Richard Rohr, Esther Myers, and Jnani Chapman.

Thanks to literary agent Andrea Hurst, editor Brandon LaFave, and our publisher, New Page Books, for making this book a reality.

And to the Great Mystery, we bow.

Disclaimer

Contents

Foreword

BY DR. ANDREW WEIL

For the past 40 years, I've focused my medical practice on developing an integrative approach to health that emphasizes the body's innate ability to adapt, change, and heal. Integrative medicine takes account of all aspects of the individual—mind, body, spirit—and how they function in unity. Medical providers best influence the health of patients by stimulating the natural capacity to heal on all levels. This capacity can be protected and enhanced through optimal diet and wise lifestyle choices, as well as by discerning use of both conventional and alternative therapies of scientific value.

As consumer interest in and demand for integrative medicine have increased, the medical education system has responded by providing more training in this area. Multiple programs and organizations exist to support the transformation of healthcare from a provider- and procedure-focused system based on curing disease to a relationship-centered service with an orientation toward healing. This does not mean that we will abandon the appropriate use of lifesaving technology. On the contrary, this innovative approach to medicine will incorporate the best conventional methods into a broader system.

I founded The Program in Integrative Medicine at the University of Arizona in 1994 to train a new breed of doctors with a deeper understanding of self-healing. That Program is now a Center of Excellence at the University and has graduated almost 1,000 integrative medicine physicians from all fields and specialties. They are in practice in all states and in many countries throughout the world. Dr. Matt Mumber is one of our first and most distinguished graduates.

It has been my long-term interest to develop healthcare systems that encourage the individual's responsibility to prevent illness and reverse disease conditions. Two of my books contain the word *spontaneous* in their titles, including the recent *Spontaneous Happiness*. The word comes from the Latin *sponte*, meaning "of one's own free will," or "voluntary." In this context, *spontaneous* describes the natural processes that arise from internal resources and without external stimulus. All of us have an innate capacity for healing. Spontaneous healing comes from within as the natural outcome of a living system in balance. To maintain optimal health, we need to trust the wisdom of the body and its capacity for self-healing, and, when necessary, seek the help of doctors who honor practices and recommend treatments that are grounded in the healing power of nature.

As the popularity of integrative medicine has grown, curiosity has increased about lifestyle measures and specific approaches that can sustain health and prevent illness. In *Sustainable Wellness*, Dr. Matt Mumber and coauthor Heather Reed guide readers on a healing journey. The authors provide just the kinds of information people need to develop healthy practices throughout their lifetime and maximize their innate healing power.

Sustainable comes from the Latin *sustinere* (*tenere*, "to hold"; *sus*, "up") and means "to maintain, support, endure." It's often used in the context of environmental issues and how we give back to the natural world. Environmental sustainability requires using our resources wisely, taking into account all the factors involved, from as many perspectives as possible. This same way of thinking can be applied to our own health.

The practices described in *Sustainable Wellness* combine a focus on personal transformation through lifestyle choices and the use of health-promoting tools. Qualities of awareness facilitate this transformation; cultivating them allows us to view life with a fresh perspective and to address small imbalances before they overwhelm our capacity to heal. An integrative approach expands awareness by looking at all factors involved in health and addressing them through the mind, body, and spirit. This broader view will help readers remain open to all approaches that support and stimulate their inner healing abilities.

Sustainable Wellness describes a larger medicine, one that includes the tremendous healing power rooted in the natural world and our own internal resources. This is the next step in the evolution of healthcare. *Sustainable Wellness* offers an approach that is practical and accessible to all.

Preface

CREATING THE CONTAINER

*W*e welcome you on your personal journey toward sustainable wellness. We've structured this book to help you every step of the way and to act as a bridge for us to work directly with you. To use a visual analogy, we're inviting you to a beautiful setting in nature and are laying out a large picnic blanket on the banks of the river of your life. We have access to a cornucopia of healthy living tools, but the picnic blanket is clean, grounded, and currently empty. We have no idea what you'll decide to place on the blanket, but we're confident that whatever you choose will allow you to live a happier and healthier life.

Approach this book and the practices it provides with gentle curiosity and openness. Try things out for yourself. When something works for you, continue practicing it. If you ever find that a tool or practice is no longer working for you, feel free to explore some of the other options and exercises.

How to get the most out of your healing journey

The information in each of the following chapters offers several resources for reflection. We've included personal experiences from Dr. Matt and Heather to illustrate this material. Otherwise the book is written from the "we" perspective with both of us speaking directly to you. Any experiences from group participants or patients are reprinted with their permission, and their names have been changed in order to maintain confidentiality. This sharing is similar to what comes up during group sessions.

Each chapter will focus on a particular area of wellness. You'll find pertinent inspirational quotes and exercises presented for daily practice. These exercises include specific and general techniques, ideas, processes, questions, tests, and explorations. Each section ends with a review of the material and specific practices that you can drop into your day-to-day routine. We call these Yoga Bits, and they are denoted by the leaf symbol. We invite you to turn over a new leaf through these simple practices.

What you put into this journey is in direct proportion to the benefit you receive. If you read this book seeking information only, it will serve as a useful resource. However, if you embrace the book's full spectrum of daily practice, the effects of self-understanding, insight, and improved physical health can be truly life-changing and sustainable. This book is not a fountain of youth; rather, if you drink fully of the practices described, it is a fountain of fully living youth, middle age, old age, and death—all of the natural parts of life.

Options for the process

You can follow this program as an individual or in groups. Your group can meet in person or online. On our Website, *www.sustainablewellnessonline.com*, you will find further resources, practices, and ways to stay connected with Dr. Matt and Heather. This site will enable the authors to work with you as facilitators. Approaching the program with a group can offer a supportive community and a richer experience. As one of our group members said, "There is something very powerful about openly sharing your heart with another."

Working as an individual is also an option, and if you choose to do so, please take advantage of the Website resources to connect with other readers going through the process individually. Please think of the authors as a part of your small group or support team. We are with you, keeping the picnic blanket in place and making sure it's able to hold whatever you bring to it.

If you choose a group setting, we recommend that you establish criteria for membership. For example, our work has focused on small groups of individuals with similar experiences because the shared experience of specific life events creates a common language that is difficult for others to understand. We worked initially with cancer patients and physicians; however, you may wish to have your group focus on specific scenarios: cancer survivors, people with diabetes, people working in the same field (doctors, nurses, lawyers, social workers, factory workers, coworkers, and so on).

If you're working with a group, we suggest meeting one to two hours a week for eight weeks—one week for each step. We recommend a group size of six to no more than 14 people so that everyone has a chance to share and contribute during each meeting. Once the group starts, no new members should join until the next group begins. This helps reinforce a shared weekly progression such that everyone is working on the same material together. This also allows everyone in the group to broaden their perspective of how specific individuals experience the same exercises, and it can offer a great deal of personal insight into what works, what doesn't work, and why. More importantly, this continuous shared experience builds community and encourages an atmosphere of comfort and confidentiality among members. If you continue the process with others who have also gone through it once before, the group can have a more open format, allowing drop-ins whenever support is needed.

It's a good idea to have two group facilitators, but they do not need to be individuals with special training in psychology or group dynamics. The facilitators are responsible for managing logistics and running meetings. The facilitators are also responsible for making sure that the basic rules and agenda are followed so everyone's voice is heard. Please refer to the group checklist in the Resources section (see page 221) for details on how to manage logistics.

The rules and agenda for each weekly meeting are the same whether in a group format or as an individual reader. For individuals or online groups, the weekly meeting serves as a review. By the end of the eight-week process, participants have developed a greater sense of what health means to them and a greater level of present-moment awareness. Most will incorporate a few new tools into their life practice, and they will see their life and health from a new perspective, fueling the process of growth and change.

The eight-step format

For the most effective outcome, we suggest you follow the order of tools and exercises presented in the book. The text covers eight steps, one for each week. There is no magic to the number of weeks, although it's close to the average amount of time it takes to form a new habit. It's important to dedicate yourself to daily practice. We suggest an average of 45 minutes per day, but you'll still see benefits if you choose to spend less time on the program. We'll use examples to discuss the basic tools you'll need for each week. If possible, find a quiet time and space where you will not be disturbed during your practice. Consider this your retreat space or sanctuary.

It's important to lay aside expectations of specific benefits from the work, as these can be counterproductive. Our expectations often limit possibilities and experience. We'll suspend judgment and expectations as we move forward with trust in the process. Next, we will define our goals and the unique characteristics that make this process work.

Creating a safe space

A motivational speaker once came to a physician group Dr. Matt attended and spoke about how to remain satisfied in the practice of medicine. One statement jumped out during his talk: "Heroes create safe space." We were familiar with opening up safe space during group work, but we hadn't come to the insight that this space could extend into all parts of our everyday lives.

The foundation of the process outlined in this book begins with the creation of safe space. When building a house, the first thing done, before any kind of planning or building permits can be issued, is to figure out where the plumbing leads. This involves some type of sewage system that will contain and hold clean runoff water and bodily waste. Can the soil support a septic system? Is there a sewer system in place that can be connected? How will it be held, transported, and processed so it's not harmful? The system must be able to hold whatever is put into it—both toxic and nontoxic.

Safe space includes holding all that we process, not only what we judge as good, but also what we have dismissed as bad and ugly. The two components of safe space are confidentiality and holding instead of fixing.

These principles are so important that we repeat them at almost every group session.

Confidentiality means that what's shared within a group stays within the group. There may be personal stories, life events, or thoughts that come out of this process that are incredibly inspiring, and you may feel that you want to share these with others in some way. If that is the case, everyone must all agree that these inspiring lessons can be shared outside the group, but only if they're not identified as coming from a certain group member. If you're proceeding with this process on an individual basis, you can carefully choose whom you want to share the process with and inform them of the safe space rules.

Holding instead of fixing means that none of us know what's best or right for another's situation. One group facilitator described this as a "'should'-free zone." As individuals, we mirror our healthcare system in the desire to fix problems, rather than holding them in our awareness while they mysteriously and slowly reveal their valuable lessons in time. This can also happen when we try to comfort ourselves or someone else who's experiencing great suffering. "It's all right," we say. "You're going to be okay"; "I've been there and gone through the exact same thing, and I made it through, so this is what you should do...." Rather than fall into a fixing and comforting mode, we hold what's said and what's happening in awareness without having to know the answer. Often our urge to fix another's issues reveals a great deal about our own life.

Confidentially holding whatever comes up without trying to fix it creates a safe space, and it is the greatest gift that we can give to ourselves and others. When even one individual opens one's heart and shares what's inside, it makes the space sacred. Sounds simple, right? The basic tenets of setting up safe space *are* very simple, but like many of the exercises we'll discuss, they're not easy.

Simple, but not easy. This is a good phrase to remember as you move along. Be gentle with yourself and others while at the same time being clear about your intentions. In reality, the process is simple *and* easy, once we get past being our own biggest obstacle to growth and change. Fully living life one moment at a time without expectation or judgment is the most natural thing in the world. In this way, we allow everything to become a teacher. But in order for this to happen, you must stay committed to the process.

In addition to safe space, it's important to define the logistical container for your practice. Be as detailed as possible, and pick a specific date, time, and place for your daily practice and weekly review. It's essential to have a well-defined schedule in order to help overcome the tendency to keep things as they are. Providing our own wake-up call allows us to move toward health and wellness. Stick to whatever schedule you create throughout the program.

Becoming an active participant

In our current healthcare system, a seeker of medical services is called a patient. The word *patient* comes from a Latin root meaning "submissive sufferer." This suggests that people who rely solely on doctors to fix their problems are quietly suffering, rather than taking an active role in their health. For many people, going to the doctor isn't a pleasant experience. There's a sense of powerlessness because you're relying on the doctor to make a diagnosis based on objective data and not based on what you're feeling. If there's nothing found with all of the tests they do, you're often told there's nothing wrong. This can be frustrating when you know and feel that something isn't right. You know your body better than anyone else.

The work of sustainable wellness requires responsible participation. Dr. Bernie Siegel was on the forefront of whole-person medicine and coined the term *respant* for this type of consumer in medicine. Respants will stand up for themselves and make sure that all sources of information are considered in the evaluation process. Medicine that's focused on a relationship-centered approach requires a provider and a respant in order to function.

It's also important to remember that this book is only a guide; you are the most important part of the equation. It's healthy to be skeptical, but please try this program to see for yourself what can happen. There are many variables that exist in our experience of health and wellness. These include genetics, current and previous illnesses, environment, culture, and personality.

You may wonder how much of your health is under your control, or if the approach outlined in this book can reverse disease, address illness, and maintain health and wellness. In our experience, an integrative approach can stimulate a person's natural healing capacity and increase one's ability to move toward wellness. Throughout the years, we have seen both minor and major changes occur in the medical conditions of participants. Many individuals have outperformed the statistics.

When the student is ready

How do we move forward with this process in the engaged but unattached manner that is so vital for change? Throughout the book we'll tell a good number of stories, and many of them will begin with the same main characters: an enlightened teacher and a group of students. One such story is instructive here.

There was an enlightened master who took on three very earnest and excited students wishing to become enlightened themselves. On the first night of instruction, the students were told to go out and find the master, who was sitting on the ground in a quiet spot near a small, still pond. The master sat in silence as the full moon floated above them at eye level, its image clearly mirrored in the water below. No words were exchanged. As the three students watched, the master slowly raised his hand, stretched out his arm gently, and pointed directly at the moon.

The first student was enamored with the presence of the master, and he vowed to become just like him. Surely, this great sage had figured out the path that would fit all humanity, and the student would focus on him for the answer. This student never became enlightened.

The second student examined the scene and focused on the master's finger pointing at the moon. The master had figured out a way that worked. It was the method that was most important, not the master himself. At that moment, the second student vowed to do whatever the master instructed him to do. He would practice daily and strive to perfect whatever exercises were delivered to him. In perfection of the practice, the answer would be found. This student never achieved enlightenment.

The third student surveyed the scene in its entirety—the master, the silence, the pond, the full moon and its reflection, the darkness, and the light. He breathed all of this in and breathed all of it out. He looked at the master sitting silently, resolutely. He looked at the master's finger pointing to the full moon. He realized in that moment that his goal of enlightenment was like the full moon: he could never attain it, and no matter how hard he strived, it would still float above in the sky. The master himself wasn't the answer for this student. The tools were but a vehicle that had utility, like his old bicycle. The key was where he chose to place his focus—on the full moon of enlightenment itself. He sat and breathed the full moon in and out, unattainable, yet fully his own in that moment. This flowed through him as his daily focus. His mind was like the still pond reflecting all that was around it. This student was enlightened.

Your teachers are there to serve you. There's an old saying: "When the student is ready, the teacher will come." Another part of that saying states that when you are ready, your beloved teacher will also leave. The tools that help you focus on your goals in life are important, but they can also be transient. Like a bicycle, they can get you from point A to point B, but only if conditions are right and we know what point A and B are, the mechanics are in working order, and so on. Different bicycles may suit different parts of the journey—a racing bike may not work very well in difficult terrain. The goal is more important, and even that must eventually be released and abandoned once it becomes a barrier—just another object for attainment. By paying attention to your life's balance, you will know when it's appropriate to have goals and when to abandon them.

Zen Master and Vietnamese Buddhist monk Thich Nhat Hanh presents an opportunity for retreat participants to write their specific questions and place them into a large bell. At one retreat, many participants asked the same question: "How do I become enlightened?" He stood in front of the group and proclaimed, "I grow tired of all of these questions about achieving enlightenment. You want to be enlightened? Breathe in. Breathe out. There—you are enlightened."

In the case of health and wellness, constant striving and grasping for balance could have the undesirable effect of creating imbalance and a lack of awareness. A perfectly balanced state isn't achieved and sustained. It's better to be flexible and open to the imperfections, so we can learn how to make small adjustments to remain balanced.

This book is a combination of the wise master and the finger pointing to the moon. The most important piece is what you bring to it—the goals that you set for yourself—and these will look different for every group and individual. Maintain flexibility within a safe and sacred container as we move forward. This is an adventure of a lifetime and every moment can bring enlightenment.

Introduction

Most of us know what's good for us and what would improve the quality of our health and lives. The challenge is creating a sustainable health plan that works for us. A multitude of programs, diets, and exercises can be found for almost every condition, problem, or difficulty, and many of these are helpful. Yet, how frequently do we try a new set of exercises or another diet, only to quit with a sense of failure? Constant exposure to new information can be stressful—even overwhelming. And forcing yourself into a one-size-fits-all framework of rules and expectations usually leads to disappointment. In the process of trying all these programs, we allow the tools to become more important than we are. Ironically, the most powerful techniques are neutral in nature. It's how and when we apply them that has the greatest power to affect us.

In *Sustainable Wellness*, we introduce a series of safe and reliable techniques that can help you make the adjustments needed to rebalance yourself as you move through the stages of life. These particular techniques come out of Dr. Matt's extensive training and experience as an integrative radiation oncologist and Heather's experience as a Yoga and meditation teacher. This book reflects our decade of work with people facing challenges of all kinds—including life-threatening ones. Whether you're looking for better health, stress reduction, or a greater sense of inner peace, we encourage you to explore and embrace the tools that resonate with you. Many of these techniques are supported by scientific study, and some have been practiced for millennia. They will kindle results as various as the individuals using them.

It's been our great privilege to share "a-ha" moments, and it has been humbling to witness lives transformed. After interacting with hundreds of participants, we've learned it's the familiar tools consistently applied that facilitate the greatest benefit and become our strongest allies. And we've seen that consistency *is* possible. This book will show you how. We'll share our inspirations—for example, the retired teacher who stuck sticky notes on walls with reminders to stop and stretch before sitting down to the crossword puzzle. We'll also give examples, such as the man who came to see being stopped at traffic lights as an opportunity to focus on breathing in the present moment.

A new world of health

A detailed observation of our current medical care system can only come to one conclusion: Healthcare has become disease care. We rely on highly trained professionals to fix what ails us, rather than place our focus on maintaining health. This approach demands that healthcare providers observe what's happening, and based on these observations, develop conclusions to explain and treat the situation.

Professional expertise is the guiding principle for the delivery of our provider- and procedure-driven healthcare system. The natural phenomena of life—birth, aging, and death—have been medicalized. We've relocated them to unnatural settings in order to exert artificial control over them, believing it would help decrease suffering and improve our enjoyment of life.

One hypothesis asserts that disease prevention will help move healthcare in a new and improved direction. The old saying "An ounce of prevention is worth a pound of cure" has never been more true than today. The majority of chronic illnesses that represent most of disease, such as diabetes, heart disease, arthritis, and cancer, are preventable with diet and lifestyle changes.

Most people know the healthy habits that prevent disease, but they struggle to incorporate them into their lives sustainably. Fad diets abound and the press is bloated with the next new supplement, pill, or technique that will fix our problems. Marketers have become savvier. All of the right words are used: *prevention, health,* and *healing.* These words are thrown around with little understanding or exploration of their actual meaning. Some of this marketing fosters the belief that conventional physicians and the healthcare system withhold valuable information in order to keep patients coming back for more of their services.

From the conventional perspective, complementary approaches are often viewed as unscientific. To compound the problem, complementary methods proven safe and effective, such as nutrition, physical activity, acupuncture, massage, and mind-body therapies, are prescribed in the same manner as a pill or procedure: downhill from an expert to a less-informed consumer. All of this results in low utilization, poor compliance, and loss of much of the benefit that a well-matched tool can provide.

The addition of ancient complementary and alternative medicine (CAM) tools to modern conventional techniques was initially touted as a way to bring patient-focused wellness back to healthcare. One early study published in the *New England Journal of Medicine* showed that patients in the United States spent more money out of pocket on self-directed complementary therapies than on visits to primary care doctors.[1] Indeed, CAM methods could encourage multidimensional healthcare. Many of them are rooted in Eastern philosophy, which includes looking at the whole person—mind, body, and spirit.

However, if complementary and alternative medicine methods are used with the same lack of awareness as conventional tools, the system is only marginally improved. In this case, the integration of CAM may bring a false sense of meaningful reform and pose a danger. We'll end up with a new set of instruments added to an already overflowing toolbox.

In our work with sustainable wellness, we use a powerful analogy: a toolbox ready at any time and filled with tools that work uniquely for each individual. One group participant shared that this approach freed her from all judgment and attachment to any particular healing system, and it allowed her to focus on what worked for her.

Does integrated medicine offer routes to true system reform as well as individual paths to sustainable wellness? We've used CAM methods in various group settings and in the clinic with great success. This book reflects our years of work together, our observations, and our stories. We believe that the integration of medicine that we've experienced offers a route for true and sustainable system reform. There's a way to optimize almost any healthy-living tool to better serve you. The magic isn't in the tools but in the process.

In CAM implementation, there's a loosely defined concept called "a match," or what fits you and your situation on all levels. Optimizing the experience of a healthy-living tool that matches a person to his or her needs is not emphasized in the current provider- and procedure-focused system, in which providers use their years of education to fix the patient's problem. A relationship-centered approach, in which the provider and patient are equal participants, works to make sure that there is a fit—not only with the proposed tool, but also with the provider, setting, and cost. In order to find a match, both the patient and physician must address all pieces of the puzzle; chief among them is the individual. What you bring to the situation, with all of your glory and garbage, light and shadow, is much more important than the tool. This is a foundational element in the ancient tradition of medicine.

Sir William Osler, whom many consider to be one of the founding fathers of modern medicine, said, "It is much more important to know what sort of patient has a disease than what sort of disease a patient has."[2] Every year, millions of patients see their physicians when they come down with the common cold. They're diagnosed and treated with prescriptions that address their symptoms and sometimes receive treatments that focus on the cause of the disease. Osler is saying that all of the variables that constitute a person in his or her totality—one's mind, body, and spirit; nutrition; stress levels; personality; fitness; social support; spiritual beliefs; and countless other characteristics—better define the desired health outcome than the biochemical details of the virus that caused the cold. The experience of having the common cold is different for everyone, and that experience is the most important part of the equation.

This opens up an exciting opportunity. The type of person that you are on all levels can provide fertile soil for health or disease. If the defining personal characteristics and practices of an individual are important, can we optimize these characteristics in a way that changes our biology? Recent studies suggest that we can. One study of comprehensive diet and lifestyle changes in men with early-stage prostate cancer showed that simple alterations could impact their immune system to better battle the cancer compared to patients who did not participate.[3] Interestingly, this same study showed that making changes in the way we live can alter the structure and function of our genetic material. In other words, the adoption of healthy-living tools can alter our genes![4]

A sustainable approach to health should be practical and should fit into everyday situations. Our actions reflect our inner nature, and vice versa: Consistent choices made over time can influence this inner nature and its expression. This is the work of transformation via the use of well-chosen tools. Small changes can have a big impact on our lives. Heather describes this through an experiment she did as a child:

As a little girl, I wandered through summer fields of wildflowers. Queen Anne's Lace was always my favorite. I wondered how the rain got into the tiny white petals and asked my father to explain. He said the flowers would show me. We picked a bunch of lacey flowers and placed them in a jar of water. My father asked me to choose among the small vials of food coloring in the kitchen cupboard and to squeeze a few drops into the water. I saw the water turn blue and asked what would happen next. He smiled and said, "You'll see." I watched the flowers throughout the day. By the next morning it had happened: the tinted water had traveled up the flower stems. The petals were blue!

Later, I learned the science behind the flowers' transformation. It paled in comparison to the magic I witnessed with my own eyes. Over time, the power and significance of my experiment has deepened. More than ever, I'm amazed by the effect of a few small drops.

This process is similar to creating a practical and sustainable health practice: The jar and the water represent our inner nature, whereas the flower reflects its expression in life. The drops of coloring are new tools at our disposal. When we use tools that merge with the substance of our inner nature, they are absorbed in a way that feeds our life and changes its expression effortlessly. If we use tools that don't align with our inner nature, they will not enter into the solution of nourishment. In our example, this would be like dropping a rock into the jar of water. The rock would sink to the bottom and would have no influence on the expression of the flower.

Throughout this book we'll offer exercises like the small drops of coloring added to the water nourishing the flower. We call these "Yoga Bits," and we encourage you to drop them into your daily life with intention and awareness. They're helpful in maintaining your chosen health practice and can be performed in as little time as taking a breath.

Sharing our stories

One of the most important aspects of our work is the sharing of personal stories. The river of every life is unique. We humbly present what we find to be beneficial in our work and in our lives. Please consider us guides on your journey to sustainable wellness. The choice and commitment are yours. We'll begin with Dr. Matt's path to integrative medicine. This experience is instructive, as it represents typical training for those on their way to becoming doctors. Where Dr. Matt's path differs is in his new way of looking at healthcare, a point of view that is now increasingly more common.

Dr. Matt's journey toward sustainable wellness

From as early as I can remember, I was trained to have an analytical approach to life. Church, school, relationships, and activities taught me that life was like a big multiple-choice question. All I had to do was figure out which option was the best and darken the corresponding bubble with a sharpened No. 2 pencil. Two things were certain: There was only one correct answer, and someone out there was always keeping score. This black-and-white approach to education laid the foundation for later medical training where specific procedures and prescriptions were applied to everyone having the same illness, rather than individualizing care based on a person's unique situation.

Education was a competition, and this competitive approach to life suited me well. Often, there was a distinct and linear path: Memorize or master a specific task, download that information on a test or excel in a contest, and then move on to the next, more satisfying task. Occasionally, there were moments of enlightenment, and I reveled in these, yearning for the day when my education would have practical applications for others. For example, I distinctly remember being awed by the deep implications of the transitive property in fourth grade geometry class: If $A = B$ and $B = C$, then $A = C$. It occurred to me that this principle is just as true for people as it is for triangles; we are all are more alike than we are different, right? But there was no time for deep exploration of subtleties, and consideration of these processes was left for another day when the invisible scorekeeper decided that type of thinking was important.

I have always had faith. I believe there is a plan. I recognized this plan in the world through the applied teachings of the Catholic school I attended. Reading, writing, math, religion, science—the answers were there waiting to be deciphered. But even with this naïve, idealistic view, I was practical about my future. People often told me things held close to their heart, and I liked to listen. I never considered this attribute a marketable skill, but my advisors thought that it was perfect for a medical career or the religious life. This option was introduced during puberty, and it made the choice between becoming a celibate Catholic priest and a doctor an easy bubble to fill in. I had always felt a calling of some sort, and medicine seemed to fit. So I began to focus on the science prerequisites needed for medical school.

Premedical and medical education focused on the workings of the human body, and paid very little attention to the whole person. Those who guided me into the vocation of medicine valued the ability to listen to another person in distress, but this skill was completely ignored in the process of medical education. The emphasis was squarely placed on memorizing the detailed biomechanical processes of the human body and then regurgitating that information on multiple-choice tests. There were many times when I thought I had made a mistake in choosing to become a physician, because the science was emphasized more than the people. Fortunately, several outstanding doctors—expert in both the science and the art of medicine—became mentors.

Then, the holistic health movement produced authors who served as examples that medicine could be about the service of the whole person and not just biology. I started medical student support groups and wrote about the narrow scope of medical education, hoping to reform the system. I also began to educate myself about what they weren't teaching in medical school. This search included how to be a doctor in a relationship with another person, and how to care for myself in order to avoid becoming a distant and cynical medical mechanic. There was a whole world of health-related interventions that were not even mentioned in medical school, and, one by one, I investigated as many as possible. I was my first patient. To this day, I continue this approach, researching potential health practices and trying them myself before I recommend them to others. I became my own laboratory for the practice of whole person–based medicine.

Residency training in radiation oncology brought an even more specialized focus: detailed education concerning cancer as a disease and all of the nuances of radiation treatment. Much to my surprise, a focus on supporting the whole person with cancer was not included during that training, and I was advised to avoid this softer side of medicine and just continue learning the massive amount of science involved in the field of radiation oncology. Well-intentioned teachers said, "When you get out of training, you can then begin to treat people how you think they need to be treated." I continued my private, whole-person education while excelling in the scientific world of radiation oncology.

Around that time, the concept of focusing on complementary and alternative medicine (CAM) was beginning to pick up steam. I attended a conference concerning how to integrate CAM and conventional medicine, and one of the speakers was Dr. Andrew Weil. Following his talk, I asked him how to best begin the process of integration. He suggested that I enroll in his newly formed Associate Fellowship in Integrative Medicine at the University of Arizona. There were 40 other physicians in this inaugural class who wanted to be more than just mechanics. The fellowship was transformative and affirmed all that I had been struggling to create on my own.

As part of the experience the fellowship provided, I attended a retreat at Commonweal, a nonprofit organization in Bolinas, California, to learn how to run residential retreats for cancer patients and physicians. They taught us how to facilitate a retreat with individuals who share similar personal experiences. We practiced Yoga, meditation, and creative writing, and told our life stories, all of which would provide the foundation for future work. Through a Yoga teacher at Commonweal, I met Heather Reed, the coauthor of this book. Heather led the Yoga sessions for our retreats and also served as a facilitator. We began offering residential retreats for cancer patients and physicians using Commonweal as a model. Dr. Rachel Remen, director of the Institute for the Study of Health and Healing at Commonweal, suggested we start slowly and grow organically, and this was our approach. In addition to retreats, our work gradually grew into an eight-step program, bringing this approach to a wider audience.

Moving forward

Dr. Matt's experience reveals one of the reasons why it's so difficult to find a sustainable approach to health. Physicians are health advisors, yet they've received very little training in how to maintain health and prevent illness. The field of integrative medicine is changing the way that doctors are trained. More than 50 academic medical centers now offer training in integration, health maintenance, and disease prevention. Countless teachers, patients, and mentors have contributed to this developmental process by showing up, speaking their truth, and sharing their experiences. Along the way, participants have learned the value of holding a safe space for themselves and others to explore new life practices. This realization opened up possibilities for personal transformation. It's the ability to see with new eyes that fuels sustainable health. The specific tool that facilitates transformation is different for everyone, but there is a process that will encourage its discovery.

Remember Heather's story about the food coloring and the flower? Well, there's a second part to the story of how the food coloring changed the outer expression of the flower. After a recent residential retreat, we were cleaning up the retreat center. We carried a vase that appeared pink over to the sink to empty the water. When we emptied it, we were surprised to find that the previously clear water had been turned pink. Further investigation revealed that there were pink daisies in the flower bunch. The dye used to color these daisies had filtered into the water of the vase, changing its color. This brought our flower metaphor full circle: Our expression of life influences our inner nature, and that inner nature also affects all of the other flowers in our life's vase. It's a two-way street. We can intentionally add new tools that transform our own life while being aware that our presence affects everyone around us. We may not be in control of all aspects of our life, but we do have free will and the power of choice.

Let's move forward together.

DEFINING
HEALTH
AND
WELLNESS

*L*ife is a constant series of adjustments; it flows like a river, swelling with rain and receding with drought, with its banks reshaping in time. The riverbed's arrangement of rock and stone re-forms in response to the changes in season and weather. Some new patterns will facilitate a crossing, and others will impede the flow. Like a river, we humans face mental, physical, emotional, and spiritual challenges as we move through life. How we grow, develop, adapt, and resist is reflected in our individual rearrangements. Ultimately, everyone faces stressors, imperfect health, and issues of all kinds. At the same time, the world around us is always changing, with our local and global environments in constant flux. Whether due to the natural cycle of life and death, or in response to disease, trauma, or accident, our tomorrows will be different from today.

Uniqueness is our common human thread. We differ in individual combinations of body type, personality, genetic heritage, culture, and experience. Our fears and desires are just as unique. Recognizing our traits and tendencies is an important step in sustaining health and negotiating a rewarding life. Our individual choices come with consequences, some immediate and others long-term. These outcomes, combined with

41

occurrences beyond our control, can subtly push us out of balance and, sometimes, dramatically off course.

What is health?

Let's begin with a pop quiz. Which of the following two individuals is healthy?

1. A 42-year-old is lying on the couch at home with a fever after catching a cold that's been going around at work. This person has very little appetite, is unable to go about his or her usual daily activities, and has decided to stop and rest until he or she feels better.

2. A chronically tired 42-year-old is sitting behind an office desk drinking caffeinated energy drinks and eating donuts to stay awake and focused during the day. This person hasn't taken a vacation in many months and feels he or she must keep working harder to climb the corporate ladder and provide for his or her family.

The way we answer the quiz's question depends on how we define health. Is health the absence of disease, or something more subtle and far-reaching? Throughout our journey together, we'll often reflect on the meaning of frequently used words. It's especially important to do this when the words can have many different meanings. The words *health, wellness, illness,* and *disease* are important to define. As they apply to our work together, they are defined as follows:

Health is a state of balance with our external and internal environment. It's a dynamic state that can include responses to acute and chronic challenges.

Wellness is the individual experience of that balanced state we call health.

Illness is a state of imbalance that occurs when challenges come up and demand a response from our resources in order to regain balance.

Disease is the individual experience of the state of imbalance we call an illness. In chronic disease, the challenges of illness have overwhelmed our resources to respond. The word *disease* is best thought of as the sum of its two parts: *dis*, meaning "lack of," and *ease*, meaning "comfort or relief." *Disease* is experiencing a lack of comfort arising from an imbalanced state that overwhelms our ability to adjust.

When we're experiencing a state of health and wellness, we're able to meet the challenges that come to us on all levels—physical, mental, emotional, social, and spiritual. When we're in a state of balance, we can adjust to a short-term illness and prevent disease. These challenges come to us moment by moment and have both short- and long-term implications.

Back to the quiz: At first glance, most people may view the sick individual at home as being less healthy than the person hard at work in the office. But health is more than the presence or absence of an acute illness. When we take a long-term view, the person at home on the couch is recovering from an illness with the normal bodily responses to such a challenge. This person's body temperature rises in order to fight off infection, and he or she is better able to do so by resting. The individual working hard at the office may look healthy, but he or she is ignoring his or her body's need for rest. Life's challenges have overwhelmed the available resources, and this person is meeting his or her internal and external demands in an unsustainable way.

This brief example shows how our perceptions of health, wellness, and the challenges of illness and disease have multiple layers. Ultimately, our ability to make adjustments that meet short-term needs while allowing for long-term viability is a key to sustainable wellness. How do we make these adjustments in a healthy way?

Consider this analogy: Think back to a time when you were sitting down to eat, and your chair was out of balance. Every time you shifted slightly, the chair moved and tipped. What did you do? You probably didn't saw off a chair leg and glue on another, or re-engineer the flooring system to balance out the chair. Generally when this happens, we take a thin piece of paper, a coaster, or a napkin and place it beneath the appropriate leg until balance is restored. It's important to notice that the chair is out of balance before it becomes structurally unsafe and our whole dinner is ruined!

Awareness and health maintenance is very similar to balancing the out-of-kilter chair. First, we need to be aware of the imbalance or challenge. Often, small imbalances can be corrected with small interventions. Moment-to-moment awareness enhances our experience of health and wellness, giving us the opportunity to address illnesses when they first appear.

A key point to remember is that there will always be imbalances. Health maintenance is not an attainment of static perfection. There will always be challenges, and experiencing illness is inevitable. Wellness is our experience of health before our ability to respond to illness is overwhelmed. When illness is ignored, it can result in long-term disease.

When a diseased state has set in, it's necessary to make bigger adjustments. This is where the techniques and methods of modern medicine have their greatest strength and best application. When an individual is diagnosed with advanced cancer, for example, many events have led to the initiation, promotion, and growth of an abnormal cluster of cells. The body's ability to eliminate them with small changes is no longer likely. The technologies and procedures of modern medicine can manage the disease process. A concurrent approach to health and wellness can get us back to a level where the body can ward off the spread or growth of any future malignant cells through activation of normal illness-fighting mechanisms. Balance can be restored and maintained through a combination of externally imposed tools and internally motivated practices. When this is done with discernment, we can stimulate our natural capacity for healing.

The three-legged stool of health

Let's take our chair analogy a little further. Now, imagine a sturdy stool with three legs of equal length. The legs and the seat are interconnected, and the ground supports the entire stool. This image of the three-legged stool is a tool that we'll use to explore the key components of health (See Figure 1–1).

The first and most important component is what holds the stool in place—the ground and foundation for health: awareness. There's an old story of a student who asked his teacher, "What must I practice in order to become enlightened?" The master answered, "Awareness." The student then asked, "What does that mean?" And the master replied, "Awareness means awareness." The student persisted. "Well how do I get there?" "Awareness. Awareness. Awareness."

Moving toward awareness

For our purposes, **awareness** is defined as the quality of paying attention to what's going on in the present moment from an inquisitive, nonjudgmental, and focused perspective. There are tools we can use to increase our capacity for awareness, such as practicing mindfulness and various forms of meditation.

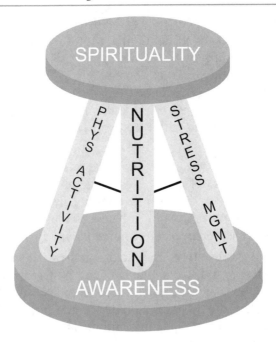

Figure 1–1. The Three-Legged Stool of Health

Experiencing awareness is like looking at a beautiful blue sky with occasional clouds floating by. When we lie down on the ground and look up, our mind usually latches onto specific clouds as they arise, change within our field of view, and then pass by. We tend to look differently at dark thunderclouds and wispy, feathery ones. Some clouds are bigger or smaller, more or less threatening. Some take on familiar shapes. Some grab our attention and we focus on them tightly, while others fade into the distance. Like clouds, our thoughts float to the past or move into the future, until we're no longer looking at the clouds; we're lost in a daydream. We may be worried or fearful about getting wet from rain or having lightning strike us, or perhaps thinking about what we did or didn't do or say in the past and what we need to do in the future. This is the usual framework of our busy mind.

In a state of awareness, all of these thoughts may arise and the clouds still float by, but instead of getting lost in the process, we're able to notice them with a gentle curiosity as they come up without attaching our mind to any one thing. Instead of identifying with our usual busy and bossy state of mind, we identify with the blue sky above the clouds. The blue sky witnesses and contains all that floats within it. It does this without any comparison to past or future events. The sky holds it all without needing to make sense of the patterns or judge them as good or bad. Awareness in this analogy is identifying with the sky instead of the busy, judgmental mind.

With awareness as our foundation, we're able to notice when our personal three-legged stool is out of balance and make the appropriate adjustments. The more we live from a consciously aware perspective, the more likely we are to notice slight imbalances that require small adjustments. Being aware is both a means to an end and an end in itself.

The three legs of the stool are linked together. They represent nutrition, physical activity, and stress management. Nutrition is the energy we take in, and it includes all aspects of nourishment. Physical activity is the energy we put out, and it includes all types of movement. Stress management is how we live with the positive and negative experiences of stress. All of these legs have an impact on the mind, body, and spirit. The stool's seat is spirituality—our highest and final concern. It's easy to see that if we aren't grounded in awareness and don't have our physical, mental, and emotional needs addressed, our highest concern in life can become focused on competitive survival needs only.

Types and stages of change

The work that became the Sustainable Wellness program began with a focus on personal transformation. Seeing things with new eyes and letting go of old hurts can balance, refresh, and renew our life. This process provides an environment in which new practices can naturally mature in time and provide us nourishment.

There's an old story about a wise sage and a renowned scholar who lived on the same street. One day they sat down for lunch together. The scholar suggested that they discuss the meaning of life, and the sage agreed. The scholar began his discourse, citing multiple traditions and philosophies, while the sage listened, smiling. The sage gently motioned toward the teapot and cup sitting in front of the scholar, asking with his eyes if he would like some tea. The scholar glanced down for a brief moment and, with a flick of his wrist, indicated that he would like some. The sage poured his own tea, and, while listening intently, started pouring into the scholar's cup. The tea reached the brim, and the sage kept pouring. It overflowed into the saucer beneath, and the sage kept pouring. It overflowed onto the table and began dripping off of the edge onto the scholar's feet, and the sage kept pouring. Finally, the scholar stopped, thinking the sage had lost his mind. "What are you doing—can't you see the cup is overflowing?" The sage gently placed the teapot on the table and said, "This cup is like your mind. It is so full of concepts and ideas that there is no room for anything new. In order to reach any understanding and insight, you must first empty your cup."

The experience of transformation is like emptying your cup. Let's use this metaphor to explore the defining elements of transformation.

- » Transformation requires space. We must empty the cup of our preconceived ideas, experiences, and thoughts in order to make space for new ones.

- » Transformation requires being comfortable with uncertainty and taking a leap of faith. When a cup is empty there is no guarantee of where, how, or when it will be filled again. It's an act of faith— of not knowing. We become curious about the present moment and we're able to sit with mystery, awe, and wonder. We let go of the need for an answer.

- » Only you can transform your life. You must empty your cup yourself.

- » Transformation is an all-or-nothing commitment. You can't empty your cup a little bit, just to be safe.

- » Transformation is often difficult to describe to another person. The experience of emptying your cup can't be explained to you as a substitute for actually doing it. Have you ever been in a group of friends when someone shares a joke that makes everyone in the group laugh, while you politely chuckle and scratch your head, wondering what's so funny? You probably ask a friend later in private to explain why the joke was so hilarious. Your friend might explain how all of the joke's parts link together to create an absurd, ridiculous, and funny situation. Still, even with a detailed explanation you may not get it.

- » Transformation is highly individual and cannot be forced on you through some distinct ritual. The way you empty and let go will be totally unique. While the basic conditions for transformation can be put into place, the process itself can't be fully defined or mechanized for a single individual. Some of our group members have found that moment of transformation in a grandchild's eyes, some in their garden, some while sitting at a stop light. Others have found it while meditating, eating, writing, or talking with others.

≫ Transformation affects every part of yourself, making all things new. The process of emptying your cup is like seeing things for the first time without preconceived notions and ideas affecting your experience.

Translational change is the type that we're most used to. It involves a specific tool or practice that's well defined, can be replicated, and has various degrees of participation. Translational change gets you from point A to point B. You can impose this type of change downhill from an expert to a willing participant. Some good examples of this are a doctor prescribing a medicine or procedure, or a person adopting a new diet or exercise program. Translational change will often be exciting and feel like forward thinking and upward growth.

Transformational change, on the other hand, can feel scary, involve facing the unknown, and feel a lot like dying to certain parts of yourself. In a culture of individuals who define themselves more by what they do than who they are, the process of transformation is seen as an unnecessary evil. Letting go of old ways of seeing and being can initially make an individual feel lost and isolated. This is one reason why it's a good idea to have support from a group of people with similar experiences.

Both types of intervention are important as we move through the various stages that define sustainable change (See Figure 1–2).

The stages of change include:

≫ Precontemplation

≫ Contemplation

≫ Preparation

≫ Action

≫ Maintenance

This process was initially described by psychologists seeking a model that would enable lasting change.[1]

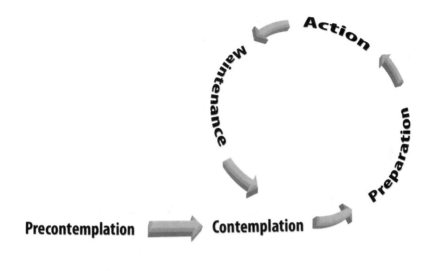

Figure 1–2. Stages of Change

Different types of change help guide different stages of change. In precontemplation, a wake-up call is usually needed to see things from a different point of view and get out of an established comfort zone. This wake-up call could be a significant or minor challenge, and it gives us the stimulus to move into contemplation. Contemplation and awareness are part of an inner journey that transformation defines. Once that inner journey has taken place, the cup has been emptied and there is space for new practices. Preparation, action, and maintenance of translational change then flow forward naturally, energized and grounded in awareness. The inner experience of insight flows into the outer expression of action. When inner being matches outer doing, a sustainable process is in place. On the other hand, when our inner being and outer actions aren't aligned, change isn't sustainable.

Exploration

Here are some questions to help you reflect on how you've made changes in the past and what has or hasn't worked for you.

Questions to ponder:

≫ When was the last time you made a major change in your life?

≫ Why did you make that change?

» Did the change come from an internal drive, or did some outside force play a role?

» How did it impact your life? How long did the change last?

Review

» Health, wellness, illness, and disease are all about balance.

» Cultivating awareness can result in an ability to notice imbalances in our life while they're still small.

» Addressing small imbalances as they arise helps maintain health and wellness, and prevents illnesses from becoming chronic disease.

» Sustainable change requires both transformation (letting go of old ways of seeing and being) and translation (embracing new tools).

» Sustainable change requires cultivating awareness, preparation, action, and maintenance in a continual cycle.

PART I

THE EIGHT STEPS TO LASTING HEALTH: STEPS 1–3

Begin Now

With decades of training, clinical and personal experience in the field of health and wellness, we know one thing clearly: We do not know. We do not know with any certainty what is good, bad, or indifferent for your unique situation. We've seen what works for one individual be totally ineffective—even harmful—for another. The best judge of what works for you is you. In this book, we'll teach you how to cultivate awareness in order to discern what's helpful and what's harmful. To begin this process, we must be comfortable with an empty cup and not knowing how or when it will be filled. Not knowing is a necessary first step in the process of sustainable wellness.

Self-reflection exploration: how healthy are you?

This exploration is designed to help you identify where you are now. Take some time to explore the following questions and statements. We suggest you revisit this section midway through the eight-week program and at its completion in order to continually remain open.

This type of work does not fit easily into answers that are 100 percent right or wrong. For this reason, we cannot develop a one-size-fits-all test that will put these questions in a format where we can score them and rate you as being at risk for disease or experiencing optimal health. Instead, this exploration is the first of many in this book that challenges you to explore more in-depth connections within yourself and focus on the quality of your life. There are definitely practices that encourage optimal health, but unlike these specific practices and objective measures, our

51

explorations are opportunities for self-discovery and more focused on personal transformation.

In order to be able to track your progress and focus on the areas that need strengthening, this exploration is designed to help you identify where you are now. Wellness is an experience of good health, and health is an experience of balance with your inner and outer environment.

There is no grading system involved here. If there were, everyone would already have an A+. The practice of non-striving, which we will discuss later, is a key part of creating a sustainable life practice. Paradoxically, non-striving and letting go of expectations opens us up to move forward with specific goals to improve our health.

1. Wellness is a state of being. How do I define my state of being and my state of doing? Can I be healthy and not well? To what degree can I experience wellness while the body undergoes an illness?

2. How do I recognize wellness in myself and in others? What does it look like? What does it feel like? How do I use my senses to determine wellness: how do I feel, sound, look, taste health?

3. How do I experience wellness as a state of balance, poise? How do I experience mind/body/spirit alignment? Is my three-legged stool of health balanced? If not, where am I out of balance?

4. How do I practice my life on a daily basis and how does that practice impact my health? How do daily health practices affect my health? Do I confuse the tool with the goal?

5. When do I begin to accommodate imbalances? Do I make a conscious/unconscious decision to ignore imbalances? Do I tend to follow the path of least resistance?

6. If life is a constant series of adjustments, am I aware of when I make an adjustment? Is it possible to live with a continuous assessment of variables? How?

7. Emotional components: Am I smiling? Am I laughing? Am I crying? Am I impatient?

8. Wellness in partnership? With whom? How would that work?

9. Is wellness an expression of responsible health?

10. As a part of your daily practice, develop a Wellness Checklist. It can include the following elements:

   a. "The Hows": How am I eating? How am I sleeping? Exercising? Relaxing? How am I relating to family, friends, colleagues? Then substitute the word Why for How.... Then When, Where....

b. List of Personal Interventions: I know that I sleep better if I walk the dog after dinner, etc. These Personal Interventions can serve as reminders, or what we call "Yoga Bits" for health, based on tendencies, personality type, genetic heritage, past experience, past ill-health, and other factors.

c. Periodically reassess your Wellness Checklist, The Hows, Whys, Wheres, Whens, and Personal Interventions.

Some individuals enjoy writing things down through the process and others like to focus on experience and sharing verbally. If you enjoy writing things down, you can begin a journal, or just scribble notes on pieces of paper occasionally in order to help focus. Reflect on your daily life practices that fit into the parts the three-legged stool of health describes. Once you have, answer the following questions: How do you currently practice living in awareness? What are your physical activity, nutritional, and stress management practices? How do you approach spirituality?

The answers to these questions may change, sometimes dramatically, as you move through the book. Recording your answers and thoughts in some format can be a practical way to track your progress through the weeks. If you decide to use a journal, the process creates a personal document of experience and reflection. Entries are written from the heart and for your eyes only. They come through awareness and bypass self-consciousness. A journal can establish a powerful reference and provide another safe space in which to explore.

Are you in balance?

Here's an exercise that allows you to see where you might be out of balance. This exercise brings awareness to how you are living your life right now and will allow you to monitor your balance throughout this process.

Exploration: Sitting down straight

Was there a time in your life, perhaps in childhood, when you were told to sit up straight? The person making the request most likely spoke with authority, if not a little annoyance. Do you remember how it felt? Sitting rigidly upright creates tension throughout the body: tightness in the shoulders, abdomen, and buttocks, the heels lift off the floor, the jaw clenches, the eyes widen, and the breath becomes very shallow. Not a pleasant experience! Yet, this is how we were taught to sit in our childhood classrooms, with holding and discomfort, much of the time. Instead, let's sit down straight.

Practice

1. Sit in a straight-backed chair and place your feet flat on the floor, with your knees at right angles. If possible, remove your shoes and socks. Take time to nestle into the chair and make any necessary adjustments to be as comfortable as possible. Invite yourself to sigh a few times, releasing your breath slowly and gently. Close your eyes, or look down toward the floor a few feet beyond your toes and soften your gaze.

2. Surrender your body's weight completely to the chair—allow the chair to support you. Pay attention to your body, as if sitting in a chair were a brand new experience. How does it feel? Notice places that may be tight and tense and, also, notice the places that may be soft and relaxed. Observe everything with curiosity and without judgment.

3. Relax your jaw and your throat. Allow your shoulders to roll back. Relax the front of your chest. Soften your belly from deep inside. Let go of anything you would like to let go of in order to become more relaxed.

4. Imagine releasing the weight of your hips and legs even more. Give this weight to the earth below. Your buttocks begin to merge with the chair seat; your feet begin to merge with the floor. At the same time, imagine the whole length of your spine extending, your neck and head extending, growing toward the sky above. Like a mountain, grounded and stable. Like a mountain, reaching into the space above. Balanced without tension. Stable without effort.

5. Continue to explore this way of sitting and being. When your mind begins to wander, smile. Bring your attention back to sitting and, once again, notice how your body feels. Be gentle with yourself.

6. When you feel ready, acknowledge your experience and complete the practice by moving and stretching as needed.

Posture influences our thoughts and feelings, and the result may be positive or negative. This is a direct expression of the mind-body connection. An association or link develops between the way the body is organized and the state of mind and emotions that follow. What we do habitually strengthens this link, often without us noticing. We can use this process to establish positive associations for our benefit. With consistent practice, a posture, like sitting down straight, begins to act like a cue. And the cue evokes a welcome state of being. The qualities of balance and stability begin to travel with us. Regardless of where you begin on your wellness journey, here and now is a beautiful place to start.

STEP 1:
MINDFULNESS

Nothing is more important than this day.
—Goethe

Moving to mindfulness

The word *mindful* is very popular right now. Many public policy–makers state that we must be mindful of where we have been and where we are now in order to know where we want to go in the future. Scientific literature increasingly reports that the practice of mindfulness and mindfulness-based meditation are successful interventions for a large variety of health challenges. With all of this publicity, there's a danger that some may see the whole process of mindfulness as the next quick fix for whatever ails a society or an individual. Quick fixes rarely work because with them, it's easier to just add new practices without emptying our cup. We must also pay attention to the quality of the container for our work. The Bible has a passage that warns against using old wineskins to hold new wine. The new wine would be ruined by the poor quality of the old container. When we are open to a new way of holding things grounded in surrender and safe space, the new practices can slowly mature. In our approach to sustainable wellness, the practice of mindfulness brings about that new way of holding things through increasing our capacity to be aware. This awareness serves as the foundation for maintaining balance.

The practice of mindfulness has been defined in various ways. In North America, the beginnings of a definition took place in a basement room at the University of Massachusetts. Jon Kabat-Zinn, a trained molecular biologist, invited physicians to refer patients for whom they had no other conventional treatment options. Kabat-Zinn guided these patients who were experiencing chronic pain and illness through an eight-week training based on his personal practice. That eight-week process became his mindfulness-based stress reduction curriculum. To the amazement of the referring physicians and the patients themselves, the process relieved suffering on several levels.

Kabat-Zinn's definition of *mindfulness* is direct and profound: **Mindfulness** is paying attention on purpose, non-judgmentally, and as though your life depended on it.[1] Mindfulness is about non-judgmental awareness of whatever comes up, without trying to change it. To use a previous analogy, it's like the sky holding all of the passing clouds without clinging to any of them.

The level of our engagement in the process is vitally important. Here's a story about the importance of commitment. One day a group of students asked their master to teach them about enlightenment. The master told them that enlightenment was like a group of men playing cards in the back of an airplane in which there were no parachutes. The stakes were very high, as the loser of the game had to jump out of the airplane. The students all immediately concluded that this game cheapened the value of life, and that if life was not valued then enlightenment could not occur. The master smiled and said, "That may be true, but think of how engaged the players would be in that game." The process of mindfulness allows us to be curious about whatever is going on in the present moment, regardless of the stakes. We pay attention to positive, negative, and neutral thoughts. It's important to realize that the stakes are always high when it comes to our health because poor choices can result in illness becoming a chronic disease.

It's equally important to understand what mindfulness *isn't*.

> ≫ It's not a religion, though the approach is a part of many Eastern religious practices, most notably Buddhism. Vietnamese Buddhist monk Thich Nhat Hanh consistently says, "It is not something to kill or die for."

> ≫ It's not trying to enter into a trance or some special state of mind. No one can impose mindfulness on you or put you into a state of mindfulness.

> ≫ It's not about trying to only think positive thoughts or distract yourself from negative ones. There's therapeutic power in using affirmations and positive psychology as health tools. There's also

a benefit to using guided imagery and visualization as methods to focus on desired outcomes and take the mind away from suffering. The ability to focus the mind into a broad awareness is bigger than these tools and is actually foundational to the successful use of any health-promoting practice.

Mindful awareness is an inclusive state of being, rather than only a rule-based system of doing. It's transformational in nature: It empties your cup, allowing space for new practices, and creates a new container that allows these practices to mature in time to take on their own unique qualities, unadulterated by concerns about the past or musings about the future. Talking about awareness is difficult because of its transformational nature. It's like a joke: Either you get it or you don't, and no one can explain it to you afterward. This is why Kabat-Zinn's work was so revolutionary: It walked the fine line of defining a practice that creates an awareness that has both transformational and translational uses. Mindfulness meditation can be both a transformational practice to empty our cup and a discrete translational tool to address specific health concerns.

How do we practice mindfulness in order to cultivate awareness? It can be as simple as breathing in, and knowing that you are breathing in; breathing out, and knowing that you are breathing out. The daily exercises at the end of this chapter will guide your health practice for this week. As a foundation, each practice session for the entire eight weeks will begin with cultivating awareness. The most important step is to experience the power of this approach.

Heather shares how she began her movement into mindfulness:

Many of my early memories involve movement. As a small child, I whirled dervish-like through the house, creating intricate dance-like patterns. Time passed unnoticed, and an audience was neither requested nor necessary. Pure joy was enough. My mother observed with interest and offered a dance class. My dance lessons continued nearly 20 years, providing a safe place for self-expression and a protective backdrop for growth and change.

Other aspects of my life were much less satisfying. Quiet and shy, I tried to follow the rules and fulfill the expectations of others. My progression through school was successful, predictable, and uneventful. While planning for college, good fortune intervened: I was awarded a scholarship to focus on fine arts as well as traditional courses. There, I had the life-changing opportunity to study movement with experienced dancers. Entire afternoons were devoted to dance, balanced with challenging academic studies in history and philosophy.

Gradually, I saw the world differently and began to consider open-ended questions, rather than calculate perfect answers. Despite hours of physical exertion, I often left the studio feeling peaceful and clear. When I danced, I seemed to move into an open, timeless place. It was possible to lose myself; worry and preoccupation would fade away. The experience was mysterious and welcome.

Once college ended, I chose a life more practical than that of a dancer. I allowed myself to shrink, and withdrew from dance. A part of me faded into dormancy. My body craved movement, however, and I was drawn to the physicality of Hatha Yoga. I began an ardent study and caught glimpses of the clarity and peace I had experienced through dance. Believing movement alone invoked these qualities, I readily pursued an intense, very linear exploration of Yoga poses. Ironically, this approach was rule-bound and full of expectations.

Before long, I found myself entangled in knots of my own making. Researching the myriad styles of Yoga lead me to a gifted teacher. During a particular day-long workshop, she seemed to sense my personal struggle and my drive for perfection. As I wound my body tightly, my teacher gently suggested that I forget everything I had learned about Yoga and instead trust in the body's intelligence. She invited me to follow my breath and to watch its wave-like movement. My response was a leap of faith. In the next breath, I experienced a profound physical and emotional release. It was joyful.

In time, I challenged the assumption that the forms of Yoga must manifest in a particular way—to be duplicated by all and immediately recognized. I realized that the practice of Yoga enriches us by accessing an internal space. Techniques are not to be learned as much as explored and used as gateways to open-ended possibilities. It is the simple act of paying attention—mindfully and on purpose—to the sensations of movement, to the subtle flow of breath, to the thoughts that come pushing into mind, to any object of focus. It is this process itself that cultivates peace and stillness. My experiences as a child, as a young dancer, as a Yoga student, were serendipitous, and once I recognized their common thread, I committed to it. In losing myself, I had found myself. Moving to mindfulness had taken me home.

Heather's story reveals that the practice of cultivating awareness can open us up to a new way of seeing and being within any set of rule-oriented doings. The magic is not in the tools or rules themselves, but in the space in which we experience them! But how do we become aware of this space?

Paying attention and becoming aware

Although there are many tools and systems that can provide a transformational experience that cultivates awareness, the practice of mindfulness is arguably the most direct. Kabat-Zinn describes seven qualities of the mind that are necessary for the practice of mindfulness. Think of a mature fruit tree. These qualities of mind are like the combination of the soil and roots of the tree. They aren't hard-and-fast rules to follow compulsively, but collectively act as nutrients to support the entire tree and the growth of a personal practice that cultivates the fruit of awareness and understanding. Much like the three-legged stool of health, all of these qualities are linked; each is affected by and has effects on the others. Often the roots and the soil interact. For the purposes of our work, we'll use the following definitions of these seven qualities of mind.

1. Beginner's mind

Beginner's mind is the ability to see things with new eyes as though we'd never seen them before. Marcel Proust wrote, "The only real voyage of discovery consists not in seeking new landscapes, but in having new eyes." We approach whatever comes up with a fresh perspective, as though this is the first time we've had this specific experience. This type of stance opens us up to the whole world of possibilities that exist in the present moment, without the baggage of automatic reactions based on past experience or expectations of future results. Although this may sound impractical or naïve, a more in-depth analysis reveals that opening to the present moment is incredibly rational.

Despite all that we've experienced in the past, and all that we expect of the future, there has never been a present moment just like this one. Instead of closing down our senses to the experience of everything that's going on right now, beginner's mind allows us to experience the totality of life, open to all that is going on to make this moment unique. It's important to understand that beginner's mind is not the same thing as letting go of all of your valuable previous experience and ideas about health and wellness. Instead, this approach means that we will look at our ideas, experiences, and behaviors from a new point of view.

2. Trust

Trust is believing in ourselves and in our authority to know our own body, thoughts, and feelings. We believe that we have the internal and external resources to sit with whatever comes up, and that the process is one that's worth following. We trust that each of us is the ultimate expert on what makes us tick and that the process of creating safe space creates a necessary support for exploration and discovery.

3. Non-judging

Non-judging is the ability to hold an open and neutral place for whatever comes up within and around you, without thinking of anything as categorically better or worse than anything else. It's a witnessing state of mind, like the blue sky holding the clouds. Past experience and future outcomes do not define what's going on in the present moment. Non-judging is a necessary ingredient for non-dual thinking. Non-dual thinking allows us to sit with mystery and paradox without needing to know the answer. This state of surrender to the present moment is key for transformation.

Dr. Matt shares a story about his introduction to non-dual thinking:

During my second year of medical school, I began a support group for medical students entitled the Group for Exceptional Medical Students, patterned after Dr. Bernie Siegel's Exceptional Cancer Patients. It was a group focused on the premise that it was beneficial for a doctor to care for patients as fellow humans, that the power of love enabled healing, and that we could support each other in learning about healing service from multiple traditions.

One of the speakers who addressed an initial group session was named Wolf, and he was a Native American Medicine Man. After his class, he invited all of us to a Native American sweat lodge ceremony to experience this cultural form of healing. The night of the ceremony, a large rain cloud settled in over Charlottesville, Virginia. Undeterred, I drove the 30 minutes to the designated site. When I arrived, I found myself to be the only person there from our group, and that the rest of those in attendance were mostly silent, preparing for the ceremony. I was scared and intimidated.

Fortunately, the clouds parted and a brilliant moon was present. Wolf walked me over to the ceremonial grounds, which were down a small hill and directly next to a half-acre pond, brilliantly reflecting the moon light. He explained the ceremony and told me that there would be a time when he would be connected to the Great Spirit, and that I would be given the opportunity to ask a question.

The ceremony was physically and mentally challenging. The group sat in a circle inside of the small igloo-like sweat lodge made of blankets and bent-over trees. At first there was complete darkness, and I could not see my hand in front of my face. After some initial instructions from Wolf, the lodge door opened and a molten red rock was lifted into the lodge and deposited in the exact center in a small hole in the ground. Water was poured over this rock, creating intense steam, which immediately filled the lodge. This occurred for several rounds defined by specific prayers and instructions.

Finally, the time came to ask the question. When my turn came, I asked, "How can I become a great healer?" The answer immediately shot back, slicing through the darkness as though an arrow was sent into the middle of my forehead: "In order to have the power to heal, you must also accept the power to kill." The remainder of the ceremony raced by as I held this answer, churning it around over and over.

On the drive home afterward, at first it seemed obvious that in order to make sure that I was going to be able to have a positive effect on my patients, I must study hard, learn all about medicine, and then I would be able to avoid doing harm and only do good. As Dr. Bernie Siegel had told one of my fellow medical students, I would need to be credible before I could be incredible. But this did not seem to fit all of the answer and I continued to look deeper. Finally, the realization struck me that healing and killing are inseparable; they're different sides of the same coin. One cannot exist without the other. Instead of being motivated to learn based on fear of avoiding a bad outcome, it would make more sense to understand the sacred ground that healing service rests upon. It's a ground that includes everything. The merciful awareness, which is brought to parts of our lives we would rather dismiss, may be difficult to embrace. Sometimes the process of experiencing transformation can feel a lot like dying. I was re-energized to learn as much as I could about the scientific and human sides of medicine, in order to best apply the tools of modern medicine guided by the mysteries of the heart and mind.

4. Patience

Patience is a willingness to continue with the process of paying attention on purpose even when it appears that no progress is being made. In the ancient Eastern mystical text *Tao Te Ching*, number 43, Lao Tzu wrote, "As the soft water cleaves obstinate stone, so to yield with life solves the insoluble: To yield, I have learned, is to come back again. But this unworded lesson, this easy example, is lost upon men." Learning and growing through mindful practice happens with time, and we can't force the outcome. It's like standing in a river: No matter how hard we move our arms through the water in the direction of the flow, we can't make the river travel any faster toward the ocean.

5. Acceptance

Acceptance is allowing whatever comes up in the present moment to be held in our field of awareness. Sometimes we may not like what we see, but we accept that the situation or our feelings are what they are. How do we accept difficult situations in life, such as receiving news about health problems? Acceptance is not the same thing as giving up or being passive; acceptance merely acknowledges that something has manifested. The opposite of acceptance in this situation would be denial. Acceptance allows us the opportunity to experience life, whereas denial pushes things away. There are times for each, and sometimes a situation is so overwhelming that denial is healthy. In defining mindful awareness, acceptance is so broad that it also includes accepting the presence of denial when necessary.

6. Letting go

Letting go is refusing to attach to specific thoughts, feelings, or behaviors. We let the clouds of our thoughts, feelings, and behaviors float by in the sky, without clinging to any one, or having any one take hold of us. This can take a lot of patience, especially when these ways of seeing and being are rooted in treasured experiences from our past or closely held beliefs. Letting go includes the ability to hold whatever is coming up in our field of awareness. In time we can begin to understand what has given life to our habitual thoughts and actions. With this understanding, we can gain insight into who we are and where we came from. Letting go can feel like losing something, but it's important to understand that every time that we say *no* to one thing, it's accompanied by a deeper *yes* to another thing, even if we are not quite sure what we are saying yes to yet. Letting go provides a space filled with calm, vibrant potential.

7. Non-striving

Non-striving is the ability to practice mindfulness without expectation of some future goal or dream. We aren't trying to make ourselves feel or be a certain way, or trying to do anything special. Emptying your cup and creating a new wineskin doesn't mean that the new ingredients will be better and more desirable than the old. This is an especially difficult quality to cultivate growing up in our goal-oriented culture of self-dependence. Here's the paradox that holds this non-dual thinking: This book is about creating a sustainable process to experience balance, and one of the key things we must do in order to create that balance is stop trying so hard to get somewhere.

A story about how non-striving can help create change is instructive here:

One day as the group was going to the store to pick up basic supplies, a student asked about the process of creating change. The teacher said, "It is much easier to travel than to stop." The students demanded to know why this was so. The wise man continued, "As long as you travel to a goal somewhere in the future, you can hold on to a dream." The students were confused. One asked, "How can we ever change if we have no goals or dreams?" The master replied, "When you hold on to a dream, you never stop and face reality. Change that is real is change that is not forcefully willed. Stop and face reality, and change will flow through you."

We have to let go of striving for specific outcomes. There is an old saying that fits: "Show up. Speak your truth. Let go of outcomes." The mindfulness practices at the end of this chapter will provide a path to cultivating awareness, when practiced with both discipline and self-compassion. These qualities of mind enable us to hold open a space for whatever comes up in life. These qualities allow us to approach the work of healing.

Healing and fixing

There is a big difference between healing and fixing. Because our medical system dominates the way we think about health, it's instructive to think about the meaning of these words as a part of the system. Our medical system very seldom uses the word *healing* as it relates to healthcare. Instead, doctors apply their knowledge to patients through technologies and procedures in order to *fix* something that has gone wrong. The only time that healing is mentioned consistently and officially is in the process called *healing by secondary intention*. This is generally used to describe a postoperative situation in which a wound can't be surgically closed due to the high probability of creating an infection. The most common example is when an injury somehow nicks the bowel, causing leakage of its contents into the abdominal cavity. In this situation, the peritoneum lining the cavity is sewn together so that all of the abdominal contents are contained, but the soft tissue and skin are to be left open. The surgeon doesn't seal it up, because it would allow for infection to gather and develop under pressure, ultimately bursting open the wound and causing a major problem. The resulting physical appearance is a large open gash across the belly. In a normal situation, this would appear life-threatening. In surgical practice, this microscopically *dirty wound* is left to heal together slowly on its own.

The word *healing* otherwise conjures up a New Age connotation. Picture images of hippies from the 1960s dancing around with daisies tucked behind their ears, gleefully singing "Heal the World." This use of the word feels superficial and flighty when compared to the graphic medical example in the last paragraph. From this perspective, healing is a magical process that requires no effort, only belief in a positive thought.

Author Stephen Levine worked a great deal with individuals going through death and dying, and he wanted to have a more personal experience with this process in order to better serve those he met. He fixed a date one year into the future and called it his death date. His plan was to live with moment-to-moment awareness as though he had only one year to live. Along the way he reflected on all parts of his life that needed to be addressed in order to be at peace. Following this experience, he wrote a book called *A Year to Live*. In that book, he wrote, "If there is a single definition of healing, it is to look with mercy and awareness at those pains, both mental and physical, that we have dismissed in judgment and dismay."[2]

This definition reveals the difficult work of healing. In order to heal, we need to look at parts of our lives that we would rather not address. In practice, healing becomes a combination of the idealistic belief in the power of healing and the surgeon's counterintuitive practice of leaving a gaping wound to give natural processes time to work. We believe in the unknown; take a leap of faith to find that what we once thought unseemly and irresolvable can actually hold great treasure. We also understand that to best serve some situations, we merely let the slow pace of time and natural processes gradually conspire to bring events to a positive resolution that we cannot clearly define. To use the non-dual language of the lesson from the sweat lodge, healing and killing are different sides of the same coin, and we cannot have one without the other.

Healing can occur when fixing is no longer possible. Healing can also make positive outcomes more likely. Throughout the years, many of our group participants have shared deeply buried experiences that had never been reconciled. Through the process of creating safe space and cultivating awareness, they were able to understand the totality of events as never before. This understanding led to compassion for all involved. Once a feeling that was buried alive is exhumed and released, the energy required to repress it is freed up. It's as if an invisible ball and chain have been released and abandoned. This energy can then be put toward living more fully in the present moment.

Stop, calm, rest, and heal

Clearly, the work we call healing is best done when we are calm, at rest, and most receptive. How do we get to a place of calm and rest in our busy lives? First, we must learn how to stop.

There's an old saying that it's important to "stop and smell the roses." There are several steps to this process. The roses represent all of life that's constantly around us. The act of smelling represents the use of the senses to engage in whatever is around us. The first step to doing this is learning how to stop. We find a way to stop our unconscious alignment with the never-ending stream of thoughts and feelings that drive our actions. When we are able to stop, we can become aware of what's going on in our body and mind. We can then become calm. When we are calm, then we can rest. When we are able to rest, then we can do the often difficult work of healing—the work of paying attention to things we would rather not address.

There's a story of a beautifully and ornately gowned prince who one day rode his glorious stallion into the middle of a small town. He stopped briefly by the side of the road, and a young boy, starstruck by this magnificent figure, asked, "Where are you going, sir?" The prince replied, "I have no idea; ask the horse."

This is the way the human mind works. The horse represents the energy of the mind and its power to influence the direction of our thoughts. Through habit, the mind has been trained to react automatically without the need for conscious choice. By stopping, paying attention, and becoming aware, there is the possibility that we can create a space between what comes up during our experience of life and our action. In that space lies the possibility of responding to life, instead of reacting based on previous programming. We no longer react like a computer program. We become aware, and then we can consciously choose how to respond. This gives us more control over how we live our lives, rather than relying on routines and hidden processes running in the background.

There's a great deal of work being done in the computing world in an attempt to create an artificial intelligence software system. Ideally, this would include a process whereby computers could learn based on previous events and develop solutions beyond a simple flow of outcomes. A simple flow of outcomes would dictate that if A happens, then B follows.

But what about the context and the myriad factors that influence whether or not B follows A? From a perspective of personal experience, when A arises our goal is to allow for a space in which a response can be chosen. For computers, the formulation is based on the totality of what can be known and has been previously translated into the world of bits and bytes. For human beings, we have a higher capacity, a natural intelligence that includes all of our senses—what we see, hear, touch, taste, smell, think, and feel. We can also practice faith, patience, hope, forgiveness, compassion, and kindness. The practice of stopping the habit-energy of the mind can result in an open space that brings the opportunity for understanding and insight to inform our choices. We can take hold of the reins of life by looking at what arises with more than just a superficial action-reaction cycle.

From a perspective of healing, this can include developing new understanding of previous hurts. Often, this new understanding and insight allows us to reframe what we previously judged as a terrible or irrevocable sin. This is an example of how the practice of cultivating awareness can allow us to heal old wounds through understanding, insight, and compassion. Witness the beauty of the seamless coordination of a horse and rider as they negotiate whatever challenges lie before them. The totality of all of the sensations and environment cannot be translated into a mechanism in order to determine the next step. Conversely, it's scary to watch a situation in which the two entities do not participate as one—each trying to exert its will over the other. How do we begin to find the ingredients that make up that seamless flow? Cultivate awareness on multiple levels of experience—body, mind, and spirit.

Daily health practice: The first week

This practice of mindfulness will be our sole focus for the first week's daily health practice. Set aside some time every day to practice. This can be done at multiple points during the day when you can introduce a moment here or there, and will be helpful in incorporating your practice into your daily life in a meaningful way. Try to set aside a formal time of at least five minutes per day at a time when you will be awake, alert, and in a comfortable place where you will not be disturbed. A chair or cushion to sit on is helpful. Begin by stating your intention to create balance in your life. Follow the explorations, practices, and reflections found in the following paragraphs. At the end of your practice, thank yourself and everyone who supported you in the process of making this effort.

Cultivating awareness is like exercising a group of muscles in order to perform a coordinated activity. Consistent repetition of a physical action, like a pitcher throwing a baseball to a catcher, creates muscle memory. Small, new movements feel much larger than they really are. With practice, the muscles all work in a coordinated flow and a personal rhythm and groove is attained. A baseball pitcher first learns mechanics, and then he can begin to develop plans for the location of his pitches. Then he can introduce new types of pitches and learn the art of game strategy. In cultivating awareness, we'll begin developing our ability to focus on something that's always available and can't exist anywhere but in the present moment: our breath. We begin by learning how to stop and focus on one thing, so that later on we can be inclusive in our ability to focus on whatever comes up. The initial mechanics will fuel the later practice of living with awareness.

Exploration: Follow the breath

Our breath is with us from birth to death. We all take a first breath and a last. This life-long process of respiration is automatic; no conscious thought is required. Inhaling, the body draws in air and keeps life-sustaining oxygen. Exhaling, the lungs release what's unusable in the form of carbon dioxide. Rarely do we notice the changes in our breathing and how they relate to the body, mind, and emotions. When given our attention, we can readily observe the differences in the way we breathe: the short inhales of surprise, the long exhales of fatigue or disappointment, and the changing breathing patterns of the body in pain or in pleasure. The miracle of breath is a constant monitor of our physical and emotional state and a faithful witness to the texture of our lives. It's the very real interface between the world around us and our internal being.

Let's explore what happens when we consciously pay attention to the subtleties of breath. What does it feel like to breathe?

Practice

1. Sit in a quiet place and take time to make yourself comfortable. Allow your body to settle and soften. If at all possible, explore this practice with your mouth closed, inhaling and exhaling through your nose.

2. Gently close your eyes and sit down straight with awareness. Let your awareness—the part of you that is paying attention—flow through your body from head to toe, and notice how each part of your body feels right now. Observe any sensations of tension or tightness. Observe any sensations of lightness or openness. Let go of assumptions and judgments about what you notice. Simply witness the process as it unfolds without trying to change or fix anything.

3. Bring your awareness to the physical sensations of breathing. Follow the breath as it flows into your nostrils and slips down the back of your throat. Feel how your rib cage expands with the inhale and your lungs fill with air. Your shoulder blades slide farther apart and your belly softly rises. Every cell in your body is nourished by your breath. Observe the exhale. Notice how it feels as your ribs softly contract and your belly rests back. Exhaling, your body slowly releases what it no longer needs.

4. The mind easily wanders. As this happens, gently bring your attention back to the breath. Be patient with yourself. When watching becomes thinking, smile and return to the breath. Even if that wandering happens a thousand times, gently bring your focus back to the breath a thousand and one times.

5. Feel your breathing rhythm and note its texture. Observe the length of the inhale and the length of the exhale. Is it the same or different? When is the breath very smooth? Where is it uneven? Observe any slight pauses or hitches in the flow of breath. Are there sensations of expansive widening or shallow restriction? Allow your awareness to ride through the inhale and through the exhale. Note where you experience the most comfort.

6. You may notice a subtle change in temperature—cool inhalation, warmer exhalation—or, possibly, hear the sound of the breath. Give the sound of the breath the same rapt attention you would give a beautiful, distant melody.

7. Finally, let go of everything you know about how we breathe, and experience "being" breathed. Enjoy the breath. Allow it to draw you deeper inside yourself. Follow the breath into a space of stillness and peace.

8. When you feel ready to complete the practice, deepen your inhalation slightly. Come back to the sensations of your body sitting in the chair and your feet resting on the floor. Very slowly and gradually begin to open your eyes. As they open, imagine looking through your eyes and seeing everything for the very first time.

Reflections

Mindfully following the breath is relaxing to the body and quieting to the mind and emotions. As we direct our awareness, breathing gradually begins to slow and deepen. The breath is always with us, and we can take this practice wherever we go. Experiment with following the breath throughout the day: during free time at work, standing in line at the grocery store, sitting in traffic, or waiting in the doctor's office. We can use regular breathing breaks, lasting even a minute or two, to reduce anxiety and soften our response to stressors. A simple practice can become a powerful tool and a lifelong ally.

Self-reflection test: How aware are you?

It takes a great deal of awareness to assess one's awareness. Are there really levels of awareness? Yes, of course; the Dalai Lama is more aware than the likes of us! We have to be careful about judgment and striving so that cultivating awareness does not become some kind of competition. In assessing one's awareness, some of the following questions may be helpful. There are no right or wrong answers to these questions. Just pay attention to whatever comes up, with an inquisitive and curious mind.

Questions to ponder:

» Can you allow yourself the space to be quiet and curious, and form questions?

» Are you willing to approach life from a different perspective, perhaps using a slightly different language? This language can include the continuum of Doing and Being, Certainty and Curiosity.

» Are you willing to see versus seek? How is the experience of seeing different from the experience of seeking? How is it the same?

» Are you at a crossroads, a pivot point?

» Has something challenged your assumptions about how life should unfold?

» Has the illusion of security been torn away?

» Are you willing to examine the organizing principles of your life?

» Can you notice patterns of thought and feelings that color your experiences?

In its simplest form, awareness comes down to dispassionate observation. That which we observe changes with each breath. In the natural world, this is a scientific fact. Physicists have proven that the elementary particles called electrons act differently depending on whether or not they're being observed. Sometimes they act as a particle and other times they act as a wave. The simple act of observation can change our nature.

Review

» Mindfulness is a state of being that can help us to empty our cup. It also includes a set of guidelines for practice and becomes a tool to address health concerns.

» It's important to nurture qualities of mind that grow our mindfulness practice in order to realize the fruit of awareness. These qualities include beginner's mind, non-judging, acceptance, patience, trust, letting go, and non-striving. These all work seamlessly together, with none more important than the others.

» Healing is different from fixing, as it cannot be imposed upon you by another. Healing can be hard work and often includes looking at things we would rather dismiss. It's best to approach healing by learning to stop, calm, and rest.

» Mindfulness cultivates awareness, which provides part of the foundation for the merciful awareness that's needed in order to heal.

» Learning how to stop and be aware of the robotic habit energy of the mind is an important step in beginning the practice of mindfulness.

» Through cultivating the mind's ability to be aware, we can develop a natural intelligence that allows us to respond to whatever comes up in life, rather than living through automatic reactions.

» The practice of mindfulness begins with developing our ability to focus on our body and the breath, ultimately allowing for the ability to hold whatever comes up in awareness.

Yoga Bits

» Pick two times during your day that will serve as reminders to stop and take a conscious breath.

» When you are walking, bring your focus and awareness to each step.

» When you are in conversation with others, take a conscious breath and listen fully, without thinking about what you will say in response while they are talking.

» Before you speak with another person about your opinion or experience, take a conscious breath, speak your truth, and let go of outcomes.

» Breathe in and out consciously while waiting in lines or for something to happen.

STEP 2:
KNOW THYSELF

What lies behind us and what lies before us are tiny matters compared to what lies within us.
—Ralph Waldo Emerson

Our first task was to commit to taking care of ourselves through a daily health practice. Ideally, you should set aside a specific amount of time dedicated to the health practice every day, possibly spread throughout the day. First, we took the time to stop and become aware of what goes on in our body, mind, and surroundings by paying attention to the present moment. This awareness can take just a few seconds and can be done at any time during the day by simply asking yourself, "Where am I?" If the answer is somewhere other than "Here, in this present moment," then you are somewhere that exists only in your mind. We spend much of our time reliving a past long gone or anticipating a future yet to come. Rarely are we fully engaged in the here and now. In doing this, our participation in life can be diminished. For some, this tendency to miss the present moment can lead to rumination and anxious worry.

The simple act of paying attention is the foundation for all that we'll experience together. It's the primary ingredient that allows this program to help you create a sustainable approach to health. This process is not like a fad diet that promises quick results only to provide long-term disappointment. It's about transforming our lives through quiet reflection, self-understanding, and persistence.

Throughout the next two weeks, we'll continue our practice of paying attention to whatever comes up in the present moment, and we'll also bring our focus to some new specific questions: "Who am I?" and "What do I want to do with my life?" It's important to maintain a curious and open mind when learning about yourself.

Exercise

Pretend that you're an alien from another planet, and you've decided to investigate this human called [your name here]. Notice what makes this human being look and sound different from others. In what ways is this human the same as others? How does he or she interact with others and the environment? What are your strongest impressions of him or her? Are there any behaviors that you would reject? Which human characteristics would you like to adopt?

Taking a more distant stance allows you to merely observe what's going on without getting caught up in judgments or the "should" zone.

Your dominant personality type

We're all born unique, and everyone has a natural tendency to respond to life in certain ways. We call this inherent blueprint our personality type. Our life experiences impact and are influenced by the way we approach life. Different people can see and react to the same life event in entirely different ways. Looking at our personality type can help us understand how we're hardwired to react. Knowledge of our tendencies can be combined with awareness to further advance our ability to make conscious choices in the present moment, rather than living life on unconscious autopilot.

Heather shares the following story:

> On a summer's day I walked a stretch of beach that had escaped a devastating oil spill. Avoiding ruin had made this place a more precious sanctuary. The wet sand cooled my feet, and the sun warmed my face. It was a walking meditation, a reverie.

Then I saw it.

A small creature launched itself out of the shallows in a dramatic arc and plunged back into the water. It happened so quickly that I couldn't make sense of it. A man started running and stumbled through the water, waving his arms wildly. He yelled, "Look! Look! It's a flying fish! A flying fish!" In amazement, I watched as the flying fish tried to hurl itself away from the shore toward deeper water. It was beautiful and strange. Its body gleamed like polished silver and its large wing-like fins were intensely blue. Its weirdness was magnificent.

Within seconds, a small crowd of people noisily entered the water. They shrieked and laughed, moving closer and closer to the fish. Several times the desperate creature tried to fly up over their heads. Why didn't the crowd—why didn't someone—move back to free the fish? Then it happened.

The net came down quickly and in one motion the flying fish was dead. After the initial shock, I felt the adrenalin of anger flow through my body. My heart pounded and my breath was jerky with tears. My eyes narrowed in judgment. How could this happen? Why?

As the crowd cleared, I saw him: a boy of 10 or so standing in the water with the net in his hand. His small shoulders were slumped as he stared down at the floating silver body. There was such sadness and disappointment on his young face. An adult stood near and gently spoke to him. I continued on my way, reflecting on my own behavior and how I had seen the whole event through the distorted screen of strong personal reaction. Who was I to respond this way? How did this happen? Why? Answering the questions brought a bigger picture into view. I hoped the boy recaptured joy, and I could only guess what brought the fish so close to shore.

So many lessons came from that summer's day. Some seem to fly out of the blue just like the fish. Others, more subtle, wait patiently in the corners of our minds and hearts. It's an ongoing challenge to trace the roots of judgments and assumptions, to negotiate the patterns of personality and behavior. But in the end, it's the unique combination of strengths and weaknesses that makes us who we are. More importantly, it gives us our life's work.

Isn't there a little bit of flying fish in all of us, our blue wings waiting to be noticed? Our quirks and eccentricities deserve acknowledgment, appreciation, and, now and then, protection. Aren't there times when we're our own worst enemy? Times when we crowd and cover the best, most vulnerable parts of ourselves? Yet with deeper awareness and gentle practice, we can find a way to move back and allow ourselves to soar.

The question "Who am I?" can result in an enormous number of answers. Roles, ancestral traits, accomplishments, feelings, thoughts, physical and spiritual attributes—all of these can enter into a complete answer of this question. All of the characters in Heather's flying fish story played their individual roles based on their personality, past experience, and other factors. For now, we'll narrow our focus to include "How do I interact with life?" as a foundational part of the question of who "I" am. We'll also delve deeper than just characterizing ourselves as having a general positive or negative attitude.

We'll explore such questions as:

- ⟫ What are my greatest fears and greatest joys?
- ⟫ What are my greatest strength and greatest weakness?
- ⟫ What attracts and repels me?
- ⟫ What are my greatest vice and greatest virtue?

An understanding of the answers to these questions is not meant to provide an opportunity to fix ourselves in order to become perfect. Instead, it empowers us to become aware of our tendencies. When we understand our automatic reactions, we can catch ourselves in the act of reacting mindlessly and allow the opportunity for conscious choice.

We use a method called the Enneagram in our group sessions to explore how personality affects who we are. The Enneagram consists of nine dominant personality types. Every individual experiences all of the types in some way throughout the course of one's life, but there is one type that is dominant for each person. This dominant personality type shapes how we usually express our highest and best self, and also how we move away from it. Our highest and best self is unified with all things and allows us to function optimally as a whole person within a whole system. With awareness, understanding, growth, and change, all of the ways that we tend to repress our highest and best self can be gradually addressed and resolved. This makes a move toward more complete self-expression possible.

Our personality can be seen as a learning tool. The Enneagram was developed as a complete and exhaustive system with many components. The full complexity of this system is beyond the scope of this book. For more extensive testing and more information about the Enneagram, please visit *www.enneagraminstitute.com.*

Each personality type is broadly characterized by the roles that the individual will generally follow. Each type contains a specific fear and desire, vice and virtue, and their specific expressions. The vices include all of the seven deadly sins: sloth, lust, gluttony, greed, pride, envy, and anger. The Enneagram also adds deceit and fear. The corresponding virtues represent the resolution of the vices: action, innocence, sobriety, non-attachment, humility, emotional balance, serenity, truthfulness, and courage.

We can use a garden-and-tree analogy to think about these components: The basic desire and basic fear provide fertile soil for the expression of the corresponding virtue and vice. These virtues and vices become the tree's fruit, and they're the primary ways that we express, or repress, our highest and best self.

Some further definitions are helpful. The **ego** is the part of us that sees itself as a personality, distinct from others, and separate from the outside world. The characteristic role of our personality type is to serve as the outward face of our ego. It's what we project to the world in answer to the question: "Who am I?" Our attachment to ego becomes a basic fallback action taken to avoid our basic fear and achieve our basic desire. Our personality type can be healthy when we are aware of it and respond in ways to maintain balance. It can be unhealthy to the degree that we react unconsciously, creating imbalance in our life while increasing our belief that we are separate beings with no connections outside of our individual self.

As we become a healthy expression of our highest and best self, we move beyond the isolated ego (and its vices) toward an interdependent, fully functioning person with virtues to share. Each type has an ego fixation, which can be thought of as the way that our separate self moves us in the direction of our greatest fear and vice. Being aware of this unconscious reaction can help us notice early on when we're moving in a direction that feeds our basic fear and expresses our predominant vice.

The Enneagram is based on a geometric figure that represents completion. An understanding of our personality tendencies can be seen as a process in which we gradually develop an alignment with our highest and best self. The Enneagram does not provide magical answers or predictions, but gives a very practical outline in which to learn that our greatest weakness and our greatest strength are usually one and the same. As such, it is a useful template that provides a broader way of looking at things. It's simply not possible to eliminate the bad and replace it with the good exclusively. Rather, our responses to life come from a continuum of countless options.

When we are in balance, our response to life will be fed by our greatest desire and will express our virtues. When we are out of balance, despite our best efforts, we'll respond to life through our vices, fed by our greatest fears. A deeper understanding of our personality type and tendencies can show us when our life is out of balance and give us the opportunity to make new choices, grow, and change.

One of the main criticisms of most personality tests is the way they tend to pigeonhole people into certain categories and emphasize what's wrong with them. The Enneagram avoids this by including states of experience. An example of a state of experience is our dominant personality type, or the culture in which we were raised. It also includes stages of development, as the expression of our personality type differs depending on the stage or level of alignment with our highest and best self. At the lowest stage of alignment we express our fears through vices, and at the highest, we express our desires through virtues. There is always room for self-understanding, and there's nothing inherently wrong with you throughout the continuum.

Please see Table 2–1 on the following pages for the Enneagram personality types and descriptions as published by Don Richard Riso and Russ Hudson in *Understanding the Enneagram: The Practical Guide to Personality Types.*[1] Riso and Hudson also published *The Wisdom of the Enneagram*[2], which we use as a guide in group settings. The Quest (Quick Enneagram Sorting Test) is a brief questionnaire that can help you to identify your dominant personality type. It's correct most of the time, but occasionally more extensive testing is required and can be found at *www. enneagraminstitute.com.* We recommend starting with the test offered here. If the results don't feel quite right, consider taking the test available on the Website for free or an expanded one for a small fee.

Type	Characteristic role	Basic Fear	Basic Desire	Vice/Passion	Virtue	Ego fixation
1	Reformer	Being bad, corrupt, unredeemable	To be aligned with the Good, the Sacred; to be virtuous	Resentment (traditionally anger)	Serenity	Judging (traditionally resentment)
2	Helper	Being loveless, unloved	To feel love, to be a source of love	Pride	Humility	Ingratiation (traditionally flattery)
3	Achiever	Being worthless and deficient	To feel valuable and worthwhile	Vanity	Truthfulness, authenticity	Deceit (traditionally vanity)
4	Individualist	Having no identity or personal significance	To find my true self and my personal significance	Envy	Equanimity (emotional balance)	Fantasizing (traditionally melancholy)
5	Investigator	Having no ability to know what's real and true	To understand reality, uncover the essence of things	Avarice	Non-attachment	Retention (traditionally stinginess)

6	Loyalist	Being without orientation, lost, without support and guidance	To find real ground and direction, a trustworthy orientation	Faithlessness	Courage	Worrying (traditionally cowardice)
7	Enthusiast	Deprivation and being trapped in emotional pain	To be happy, free, and satisfied; fulfilled	Gluttony	Sobriety	Anticipation (traditionally planning)
8	Challenger	Being destroyed, lifeless, violated	To feel strong, real, and alive	Lust (forcefulness)	Innocence	Objectification (traditionally vengeance)
9	Peacemaker	Loss of my world, disconnection, being cut off, fragmentation, separation	Wholeness, inner stability, peace of mind	Sloth (disengagement)	Engagement	Ruminating (traditionally indolence)

Table 2–1. Enneagram Personality Types. The Riso-Hudson QUEST (SM)—The Quick Enneagram Sorting Test (*The Wisdom of the Enneagram*, Don Richard Riso and Russ Hudson, pp. 14–18. Reprinted with permission from Riso-Hudson.)

Instructions

For the QUEST to yield a correct result, it is important that you read and follow these few simple instructions.

» Select *one* paragraph in each of the following two groups of statements that best reflects your general attitudes and behaviors, as you have been most of your life.

» You do not have to agree completely with every word or statement in the paragraph that you select. You might agree with only 80 or 90 percent of a particular paragraph and still select that paragraph over the other two in the group. However, you should agree with the general tone and overall "philosophy" of the paragraph that you select. You will probably disagree with some part of the paragraphs.

» Do not overanalyze your choices. Select the paragraph that your "gut feeling" says is the right one for you, even though you may not agree with everything it says. The general feeling of the paragraph as a whole is more important than individual elements of it. Go with your intuition.

» If you cannot decide which paragraph best fits you in one of the groups, you may make two choices, but only in one group; for example, *C* in Group I and *X* and *Y* in Group II.

» Enter the letter you have selected for that group in the appropriate space following Group II.

Group I

A. I have tended to be fairly independent and assertive: I've felt that life works best when you meet it head-on. I set my own goals, get involved, and want to make things happen. I don't like sitting around; I want to achieve something big and have an impact. I don't necessarily seek confrontations, but I don't let people push me around either. Most of the time I know what I want, and I go for it. I tend to work hard and play hard.

B. I have tended to be quiet and am used to being on my own. I usually don't draw much attention to myself socially, and it's generally unusual for me to assert myself all that forcefully. I don't feel comfortable taking the lead or being as competitive as others. Many would probably say that I'm something of a dreamer; a lot of my excitement goes on in my imagination. I can be quite content without feeling I have to be active all the time.

C. I have tended to be extremely responsible and dedicated. I feel terrible if I don't keep my commitments and do what's expected of me. I want people to know that I'm there for them and that I'll do what I believe is best for them. I've often made great personal sacrifices for the sake of others, whether they know it or not. I often don't take adequate care of myself; I do the work that needs to be done and relax (and do what I really want) if there's time left.

Group II

X. I am a person who usually maintains a positive outlook and feels that things will work out for the best. I can usually find something to be enthusiastic about and different ways to occupy myself. I like being around people and helping others to be happy. I enjoy sharing my own well-being with them. (I don't always feel great, but I try not to show it to anyone!) However, staying positive has sometimes meant that I've put off dealing with my own problems for too long.

Y. I am a person who has strong feelings about things. Most people can tell when I'm unhappy about something. I can be guarded with people, but I'm more sensitive than I let on. I want to know where I stand with others and who and what I can count on. It's pretty clear to most people where they stand with me. When I'm upset about something, I want others to respond and to get as worked up as I am. I know the rules, but I don't want people telling me what to do. I want to decide for myself.

Z. I tend to be self-controlled and logical. I am uncomfortable dealing with feelings. I am efficient—even perfectionistic—and prefer working on my own. When there are problems or personal conflicts, I try not to bring my feelings into the situation. Some say I'm too cool and detached, but I don't want my emotional reactions to distract me from what's really important to me. I usually don't show my reactions when others "get to me."

Group I choice: _____
Group II choice: _____

Together the two letters you have selected form a two-letter code. For example, choosing paragraph *C* in Group I and paragraph *Y* in Group II produces the two letter code *CY*. To find out which basic personality type the QUEST indicates you are, see the following QUEST codes.

2-Digit Code	Type	Type Name and Key Characteristics
AX	7	The Enthusiast: Upbeat, accomplished, impulsive
AY	8	The Challenger: Self-confident, decisive, domineering
AZ	3	The Achiever: Adaptable, ambitious, image-conscious
BX	9	The Peacemaker: Receptive, reassuring, complacent
BY	4	The Individualist: Intuitive, aesthetic, self-absorbed
BZ	5	The Investigator: Perceptive, innovative, detached
CX	2	The Helper: Caring, generous, possessive
CY	6	The Loyalist: Engaging, responsible, defensive
CZ	1	The Reformer: Rational, principled, self-controlled

Table 2–2. QUEST Code Results

Your dominant personality type is the way that you generally interact with the world. You do not pick it out and cannot choose a different type because it seems more appealing. Knowing your greatest fear and greatest desire can help you catch yourself in the act when you apply your awareness to your ways of being and doing. Understanding your general tendencies can help you find balance in all aspects of your life.

Once you have identified your dominant personality type, it's time to put on your alien investigator helmet! Try the following exercise in order to explore this process further.

Exploration: Where am I coming from?

Usually, we don't see the world the way it is; we see the world the way we are. Our personality type, along with everything that makes us unique, becomes an interface with our world. Each one of us develops a kind of multidimensional screen that helps us sort and analyze, judge, and make decisions. Much like a well-used window screen, this personal screen can get a little hard to see through in time. The roots of our opinions and assumptions can become unclear. Eventually, our thought patterns can become unconscious habits. And it's always easier to judge someone else's behavior than to analyze our own.

The familiar sayings "Where is she coming from?" and "He's pushing my buttons!" usually come up when we bump into a different personality type or when we feel misunderstood. When this happens, it's easy to be defensive and reactive. Instead, let's explore turning those questions around and consider where *we're* coming from and how we got those buttons in the first place.

Practice

Have you ever noticed how we tend to sit in the same chair, in the same part of the room, over and over? How we also take the same seat on the bus each time, follow the same route home each day, and shop through the grocery store in the same pattern each week? Let's consider how our patterns and choices become so fixed and routine. What would it feel like to change them?

For this practice, find a different place to sit, with a different view of the room.

≫ Begin by sitting down straight with awareness. As you feel settled, quietly observe your surroundings from this new vantage point. Observe all that you see without judgment. Release your opinions about the room and everything in it. Notice its shape and size as if you'd never been there before. Bring your attention to the corners of the room, to the ceiling, and to the floor. Observe the space around the objects in the room and in between them. Bring your awareness to the space above your head, under your seat, and all around you.

≫ Now bring your awareness to the space within. Gently close your eyes and invite your body, mind, and heart to relax and soften more completely. Feel the physical sensations of the breath as it moves through you. Follow the breath for a minute or two. Allow the breath to lead you deeper and deeper inside yourself.

≫ As thoughts occur, let them pass by like clouds floating across the sky. Notice the space between thoughts and allow the space to expand. Stay here for a while—spacious and free. Be here and remember who you really are.

≫ As you feel ready, begin to deepen your breath. Feel your body sitting in the chair. Feel your feet resting on the floor. Slowly open your eyes. As you look through your eyes, imagine seeing everything for the very first time.

Reflections

Understanding our habits and tendencies, strengths and weaknesses, fears and desires helps refresh our personal screen. Awareness brings an opportunity to recognize and assess our patterns and knee-jerk reactions. After all, haven't we played some part in manufacturing our own buttons? With quiet reflection, attitudes can be explored and even modified. While still honoring our uniqueness, we develop a more panoramic view. And with a wider viewpoint, we might just see where someone else is coming from.

Review

≫ We are all born with a dominant personality type that guides how we interact with the world.

≫ Understanding our basic fear and basic desire can help us catch ourselves reacting automatically based on our tendencies. When we catch ourselves in this way, it gives us the opportunity to make choices that maintain our balance in life.

≫ Our personality can grow and develop in time and more positively express our wholeness.

Yoga Bits

≫ Sit in a different seat than you usually sit in during a meeting or at home. Notice how this feels.

≫ Write your ego fixation on a small index card and post it somewhere where you can see it throughout the day. If you catch yourself in the act of expressing this fixation, stop and take a conscious breath.

≫ Choose one small action to express your dominant personality type virtue or any virtue.

Step 3:
Life Review
and Planning

Life can only be understood backwards, but it must be lived forwards.
—Søren Kierkegaard

This week we'll bring our focused awareness to what our life has looked like in the past and create a roadmap for moving forward. This process takes a lot of courage and persistence; we'll need to explore the parts of our past and present that we'd rather ignore. Diligence is also needed when planning for the future so we don't require some heroic effort or sheer willpower alone to fix our lives and make them perfect. This is where trust—in ourselves and the process—comes in. We trust that our lives are perfect as they are, everything is as it needs to be, and there is still room for growth and change.

There is a way that we can move forward with courage, trust, and focus.

1. First, we ask simple questions.
2. Second, we pay honest attention to what comes up, without judgment.

3. Third, we hold open space for whatever comes up to *just be* in our consciousness without needing an immediate answer. We surrender our attachment to creating a specific outcome.

Remember that confidentially holding whatever comes up without trying to fix it is the key that unlocks the door to sustainability. This holding without fixing may seem counterintuitive to creating a clearly defined goal, but it's not. When we create a goal without present-moment awareness, without insight and understanding of who we are and where we have been, then we're already out of balance before we get started. A deep understanding of past experiences leads to the gift of discernment that can guide us in making present-moment choices.

Life review

All the world's a stage,
And all the men and women merely players;
They have their exits and their entrances,
And one man in his time plays many parts....
—William Shakespeare, *As You Like It*

The life review process can be looked at from different angles. In a near-death experience, a life review is what happens when one's life flashes before one's eyes prior to death. Those who have had a near-death experience say that this process happens almost instantaneously, and it's like watching a movie filled with important scenes from their life. Some return from this experience with a new way of seeing and being. They don't repeat the mistakes of the past, especially anything that might harm them or others. They see things from a different point of view and this transforms them. Transformational change is usually like this. It's generally a sudden change brought on by an "a-ha" moment. This new way of seeing is translated into a new way of being. This process usually takes time. The occasional difficulties encountered by adopting new ways of being are made tolerable by the inspiration gained from the new way of seeing.

Another kind of life review comes from counseling techniques used for elderly people or those facing terminal illness. In this setting, a group of questions are presented in order to form a life summary. An individual can use this practice as a method to integrate life experiences in a way that resolves old grievances, celebrates accomplishments, and passes on their legacy to ancestors.

Our journey together includes looking at ourselves as whole beings. The ultimate integrative system is best described by Ken Wilber, in his book *A Brief History of Everything.*[1] An integrative approach must include looking at all participants at all levels of their being and experience.

Let's look at this integrative approach one part at a time.

1. All participants. Anyone who has had an impact on our lives should be included in this category. Sometimes just opening up our lens to see that people—with whom we never personally interacted—had a major impact on our lives, can lead to new understanding.

2. All levels of being. When we look at all levels of being, we include who we are spiritually, mentally, emotionally, and physically.

3. All levels of experience. All participants experience these levels of being through multiple filters. These filters include the lenses of the self, culture, and the natural world.

   ≫ The lens of self. The previous chapter focused on how the filter of our individual dominant personality type can affect how we interact with the world.

   ≫ The lens of culture. Different cultures also have dominant personality characteristics that can influence how well individuals fit in to the society in which they live. For example, an aggressive, achievement-oriented individual would be more of a match for the predominant culture of the United States than that which was traditionally associated with Eastern cultures such as China and India. Of course, cultures can change their predominant personality type in time, as we have seen with Eastern cultures becoming more aggressive and achievement-oriented.

   ≫ The lens of the natural world. The natural world has a major impact on how we live. The presence or absence of basic necessities, living in urban or rural settings, being exposed to natural disasters or insulated from them, and so on—these features affect how we interact with our natural surroundings. As individuals we have a major impact on the natural world by our actions, how we consume resources, and how we replenish the environment.

If we were to leave out any of these important factors, we would have an incomplete picture of the whole situation. Understanding the complete picture of our life relative to all participants at all levels of seeing and being is preferable when we want to be fully present and move forward in a sustainable way.

When you become aware of any significant event in life, you'll have the opportunity to learn from it. An integrative perspective broadens your field of awareness and helps complete your understanding. An integrative perspective is an important complement to an awareness that is as expansive as the blue sky and able to hold anything.

Life review process

For the life review categories presented in the paragraphs following the short Awareness Exercise, we recommend writing in a journal that you can return to whenever a new insight or memory comes along. If you prefer not to put things in writing, we recommend that you contemplate each set of questions one at a time. Perhaps you could review one category per day. In either case, first read through all of the categories presented here to get a broad overview of the entire landscape. Then go back and begin with the first set of questions. Answering the questions is more like creating a piece of artwork than solving a puzzle. Once you've gone through all the categories, you may want to put it aside to read later as if it were another person's life story. You could also choose to act on any new insights you've gained.

Awareness Exercise:

Stop, Calm, and Rest

Begin each period of integrative life review with a simple awareness exercise such as this in order to stop, calm, and rest while approaching this healing work.

Ask yourself "Where am I?" Don't begin until the answer is "In the here and now."

If you find that recalling events drags you away from the present moment, return to it with the experience of breathing. You can focus on the breath with this exercise, inspired by Vietnamese Zen Master Thich Nhat Hanh.[2] It is a good one to help train the mind to hold a specific focus. When your mind wanders—and it will—bring your focus gently back to the breath. The breath is a wonderful practice anchor, because it can only exist in the present moment. Then, you can bring your attention back to the current point of focus. This wandering of the mind may happen over and over, and does not mean that it was a bad performance of the exercise. When our mind wanders, we bring the focus back with persistence and gentleness.

Either think or say aloud:

I stop the momentum of the day, with nothing to do and nowhere to go.

Nothing to do and nowhere to go.

I bring my focus to the breath, wherever I feel it the most in my body—it could be at the nose, in the chest, or in the belly.

Breathing in and breathing out.

Just breathing.

[Pause for four breaths.]

I enjoy the feeling of breathing in and out.

Enjoying.

[Pause for four breaths.]

I notice my whole body and see that it has become more calm.

Calming.

[Pause for four breaths.]

As I enjoy my breathing, I rest.

Resting here and now.

[Pause for four breaths.]

I can now place my calm focus wherever I would like.

Category 1: Participants

In this section, you'll consider individuals who've had an impact on your life. While sitting with your thoughts and feelings about these players on the stage of your life, try to remember as many details as possible. If there are specific individuals who've had major impact, positive or negative, you may wish to explore what you know or can learn about their individual levels of being (body, mind, and spirit) and experience (their personality, their culture, and the natural world in which they live[d]). This may lay the ground work for understanding their actions. As you review all of these questions, think about or write down whatever initially comes to mind without trying to further understand it. At a later date, bring your focused attention to what has come up with the goal of understanding how these details of your life have impacted who you are today and how you make your choices.

Family

List your immediate and extended family. Include as many people as possible, as far back as you can go, whether you ever met them or not. Brothers and sisters, fathers, mothers, step-relations, grandparents, great-grandparents, great-great-grandparents, aunts and uncles, cousins, your spouse, in-laws, children, grandchildren, great-grandchildren, and so on.

Questions to ponder:

» Which of these individuals had the greatest impact on you?

» What is your first memory of your father or mother? Answer this question for all relatives who made an impression on you.

» What are the most important events that you recall associated with your family members?

» What is your most enjoyable family-related memory?

» What is your most distressing memory?

» What did your family teach you—either as individuals or as a whole?

» How has your family shaped who you've become?

» Was there anyone you particularly identified with?

» Do you hold any family grievances? If so, what events surrounded the creation of those grievances?

Friends

List as many friends as possible from as far back as you can remember.

Questions to ponder:

» Who was your first best friend?

- How did you meet?
- What did you do with him or her?
- What was your relationship like?
- Do you tend to have many superficial friendships, or intense relationships with one or two friends?
- How do you choose your friends?
- What are the most important events you shared with friends?
- If there was one event you shared with friends that you could live again, what would it be? Why?
- What was the most exciting event you shared with a friend(s)?
- What was the most satisfying?
- What was the most distressing?
- Are there any old grievances?
- Are there any friends you've lost touch with?
- Are there any friends who've become enemies? If so, how did that happen?

Mentors

List as many mentors as possible from as far back as you can go.

Questions to ponder:

- How did you connect with these individuals?
- Did you meet?
- What important lessons did you learn?
- How did your mentors teach you? Was it through stories, examples, or discussions?
- What type of teaching affected you the most?
- Are there any mentors who disappointed you in some way?
- What is the most important lesson you learned from a mentor?
- Is there something a mentor taught you that made no sense at first but later rang true?

Acquaintances

List as many acquaintances as you can remember.

Questions to ponder:

» Can you remember any distinguishing characteristics of these individuals?

» What kept them on the periphery of your life?

» Did any initial acquaintances become friends?

» Are there any events that you shared mainly with acquaintances?

Other

List other people who have had an influence on your life. These could include famous people from your lifetime or throughout history.

Questions to ponder:

» How did these individuals affect you? Was it in a positive or negative way?

» Was it through their writing, their actions, or others teaching you about them?

» Who had the greatest effect, and why?

Category 2: Levels of being

The levels of being include a present-moment awareness of everything happening in our mind, body, and spirit. Our normal habit energy rules the things we usually do automatically in reaction to a situation. This habit energy often restricts our experience to reacting only to the predominant process occurring right now without any understanding of the situation or any ability to choose a response. It's almost as though we get stuck in survival mode. In this mode, we react instantaneously based on previous conditioning, dominant personality type, and our expectations of future results. We react first and ask questions later. There are some situations in which this is vital—such as when we're standing in the middle of a road and a speeding car is approaching. But unlike survival mode, most situations in life benefit from a responsive approach, which can include conscious choice.

In understanding our past levels of being, we have the present-moment advantage with our ability to stop, calm, and rest. Then we can reflect on past processes that we dismissed as too difficult to address while we experienced them. As we witness past events non-judgmentally, we may get a "be over" instead of a "do over." We can take our calm, responding, present-moment self back to a past experience. Now, we can "be" the experience in a state of calm and rest, when before we were involved in the immediate drama and could only unconsciously and reactively "do" it.

When revisiting past events, we obviously can't change the way we acted, but we can bring new levels of understanding and insight to situations that cause old hurts that exist to this day. In this way, we can recognize parts of ourselves that we had previously dismissed. By doing so, we can recover our wholeness. We bring our present-moment awareness to the past in a way that helps us to address balance right now.

There is a difference between living in the past and visiting the past with our present-moment awareness. When we live in the past, we miss the present moment and are distracted and reactive. Many of our group participants have realized the significant benefit of bringing forgiveness and understanding to past experience through a more whole and inclusive present moment. Ultimately the key to looking at difficult thoughts, events, or experiences can be summed up simply: We can witness. When thoughts carry us away, we can remember to hold space for them without judgmental attachment, and use the breath as an anchor in the present moment.

Imagine a very tall tree in a storm. The tree's upper limbs move about wildly, and the whole tree may seem ready to blow away with the wind. We fear what might happen and feel out of control. This is similar to our thoughts about difficult experiences. If we focus on the trunk of the tree, we can see that the tree is firmly rooted to the ground even in powerful winds. This connection is like our breath. When we get lost in the wild activity of our thoughts, we can bring our focus to the breath and become grounded in the present moment. Thoughts pull our attention to the past or to the future, but the breath only exists in the present moment. In focusing on the strong trunk of the tree, there is stability and fearlessness. This is a good place to be when we visit old hurts. Revisiting the past can also be an enjoyable experience and bring gratitude for all that life has given us. If we're alive and breathing, there is much to be grateful for. Gratitude, forgiveness, and insight can provide the inspiration to continue our chosen life practice.

Physical

The physical body gets us where we want to go and also becomes a vehicle for self-expression. Looking at how we relate to our physical self is an important tool. Mental, emotional, and spiritual gains and losses can have physical expressions. Our physical scars and attributes can be great teachers.

Questions to ponder:

- ⋙ What are your earliest physical memories?
- ⋙ Are those memories centered around pain, pleasure, comfort, movement, or stillness?
- ⋙ What are the major life events of your body?
- ⋙ Are there any that stand out as most significant?
- ⋙ Did you have any injuries or trauma? Think about the physical characteristics of these events.
- ⋙ What is your relationship with your body?
- ⋙ How do you treat your body?
- ⋙ What roles do movement and playtime have for you?
- ⋙ Picture that you are able to stand in front of the mirror at various stages of your physical development. How did you view your body during each of these stages? How do you view it now?
- ⋙ What are your greatest physical challenges?
- ⋙ What are your greatest physical accomplishments?
- ⋙ If your body could speak, what would it say to you?
- ⋙ Remember when you felt the most physically strong and the most physically weak. Describe how each of these situations felt and how you got there.
- ⋙ Remember times when you pushed your body to the limit. What was that like?

Mental/Emotional

Our mind and emotions play a major role in how we view life. We don't come into life with instructions for how to maximize the use of this wonderful resource. The practice of mindfulness can help us train our mind to notice and respond instead of automatically reacting based on previous experience and habit. It's helpful to witness past activities of our mind in order to have a reference for the present.

Questions to ponder:

- ⋙ What is the first feeling you can remember? Describe it in as much detail as possible.

>> What is the first thought you can remember?

>> Do you have thoughts and feelings that come up again and again? What are they?

>> Can you remember a time when you released a significant recurring concern? Describe how you were able to let go of that concern.

>> What were the most joyful times in your life? What were the most challenging and distressing times? Remember them in as much detail as possible. Witness them from a calm place.

>> What is your learning style; visual, auditory, sensual, or tactile?

>> Have you had difficulty learning?

>> What was school like for you?

>> Do you learn more from experience or from books?

>> What are your greatest emotional strength and greatest weakness?

>> Can you remember a time when you felt the most vulnerable and a time when you felt the most invincible?

>> What is your greatest joy? Your greatest fear?

>> What is your greatest disappointment in life?

>> What do you consider your greatest accomplishment?

Spiritual

Spirituality gives our life meaning through alignment with our highest and final concern. Our approach to spirituality may broaden in time, and different practices or tools may resonate at different times in life. Spirituality may also include how we feel connected to Life with a capital "L," which includes the whole wonderful and mysterious universe and all creation.

Questions to ponder:

>> What is your highest and final concern in life?

>> What are the most important parts of life for you? The least important?

>> What is your understanding of God?

>> Was there a time in your life when you felt especially close to God? Especially far away?

>> What role did religion play in your life?

>> How do you define spirituality?

>> How do you define religion?

>> Where do you think you were before you were born?

>> Where do you think you go after you die?

>> How do you care for yourself, others, and the natural world?

>> If you could pick a theme for your life that you would like to leave as a legacy, what would that theme be?

>> What gets you out of bed in the morning?

>> Are there areas of your life where you feel you need forgiveness for yourself or others?

>> What role has forgiveness played in your life?

>> What are you most proud of in life?

>> What do you most regret?

>> When have you felt most at peace?

>> When have you felt most in turmoil?

>> Is there any experience you carry around of which you feel guilty or ashamed?

>> What makes you feel the most joyous?

Category 3: Our filters of experience

If we only look at the details of our life from the same perspective from which we experienced them, a life review will be little more than a summary. But when we bring a sense of calm focus grounded in the present moment, the perspective changes. It's like sitting in a different spot in a familiar room. The next step is the realization that all of our experiences are filtered through multiple lenses, some of which we can't control. We can't control the culture we're born into or the characteristics of the natural world. Our dominant personality type is also something we're born with; we don't have the opportunity to select it. The more we know about the scenes in which our lives are played out, the more we develop understanding. With understanding, it's possible to gain insight into our life events. With insight comes compassion. Compassion in action includes a desire to lessen suffering and increase enjoyment of life for ourselves and others. Let's take at a look at the lenses of self, culture, and the natural world.

Self

The Enneagram system points out that we experience all of the vices and virtues that face humanity, and we also have a dominant personality that teaches us the majority of the lessons. The Enneagram also includes levels of development, through which we express our personality features differently depending on our balance and health. Generally speaking, the less we're attached to the survival concerns of our limited and separate self (ego) and the more we're concerned with embracing wholeness, the more balanced and healthy we'll be. When we're balanced and healthy, the fruits of our personality express themselves in the form of virtues specific to our type and relative to other types. The opposite is true when we are out of balance.

Here are some questions to help you understand how your personality has influenced how you see the world and the basis of your actions, both conscious and unconscious. With this understanding comes an increased ability to find balance in our responses to life. In our three-legged stool analogy, balance is found when the stool has an equal distribution and feels steady on the ground of our awareness.

Questions to ponder:

- How do you relate to the world?
- How would you describe yourself to someone else?
- How do you face challenges?
- How do you interact with others?
- What is your greatest desire? Your greatest fear?
- How has your personality influenced your choices in life?
- Are your actions different when you are balanced than when you are out of balance? Describe some specific situations in which your choices may have been different if you'd been in a more balanced place.
- How do you maintain balance in life?
- What motivates you?
- What makes you want to give up?

Culture

In this section, we'll explore how the filter of our culture has shaped us and influenced our decision-making. *Culture* can be defined as the predominant way of looking at life as a group. It forms the foundation for any group activity. We often hear leaders speak about cultural change being necessary to create change throughout a system. Usually changing a culture begins by reflecting on the present features with clarity and without bias. Understanding our cultural influences can lead to gratitude and forgiveness as well as the increased ability to make conscious choices concerning change.

Questions to ponder:

⋙ What are the characteristics of the predominant culture in which you live?

⋙ Have you lived in different cultures?

⋙ Does your family's cultural background fit in with that of the society where you live?

⋙ Do you feel accepted and at home in the culture you live in, or do you feel like an outsider?

⋙ What are some experiences that made you aware of the predominant culture in which you live?

⋙ Are there specific aspects of your culture with which you disagree or feel uncomfortable?

⋙ Are you proud of parts of your culture? Are you in agreement?

⋙ If you could change one aspect of your culture, what would it be?

⋙ Have you been involved in a culture change, even to a small degree? How did that culture change happen? How did you feel about that change? Did you participate in making it happen? Did you resist it? Are there parts of other cultures that you admire, embrace, detest, or actively resist?

Natural world

This spaceship that we call Earth has been around for many eons. We can look at Earth as something with which we've been entrusted. Many people rally around the cry to "Save the Earth." To paraphrase the late, great comedian George Carlin: The Earth will be fine; it's the humans that are in trouble. The natural resources from this planet are the source of the majority of monetary wealth that individuals, corporations, and governments accumulate. Our use of these resources literally keeps humanity alive. It's as though the human race represents all those aliens in movies who come to Earth because they have greedily used up all of their own planet's resources. Unless we focus our awareness on wise use and replenishment of basic resources, human life will not be sustainable, nevermind wellness.

The phrase, "think globally, act locally" is a nice fit here. We need to understand how we have interacted with our natural world and how we can respond in order to create an effective balance. Sustainable wellness for an individual has to include a sustainable approach for our planet. Here are a few questions to help guide the process of understanding how the natural world has impacted you and how you have impacted the natural world.

Questions to ponder:

- What are your earliest memories of the natural world?
- Do you have any memories that bring up significant fear?
- What are some experiences that have made you feel connected with the natural world? What are some that have made you feel disconnected?
- What is your most pleasant memory of being in nature?
- What is your favorite spot on Earth? Why?
- Do you have any experience of being cared for, nurtured, or sheltered by the natural world?
- What is your most joyous experience in nature?
- How have you cared for the natural world?
- How have you been a good and bad steward for nature?

Now that we have looked at all participants in our life and considered all levels of being and the various filters of experience, it's time to stop and rest again for a moment. If you've gone through this process with awareness, you may feel as though you've just given birth to a more complete version of you! Now that we've done a life review, we can step back and question where we want to go from here. Before doing so, take at least one more look at all of the material just presented.

Let's now proceed with taking our present-moment awareness into the realm of planning for the future.

Life planning

Planning is bringing the future into the present so that you can do something about it now.

—Alan Lakein, *How to Get Control of Your Time and Life*

We've investigated where we are now and also where we've been. We'll now plan for where we want to go in the future. Planning is typically one of the more difficult assignments of the eight-week experience. It tests our ability to be mindful on multiple levels.

» We can approach this process with a beginner's mind, and an openness to new approaches and new goals in life.

» We can trust that despite all of our weaknesses and past disappointments, we can make the best choices possible in this present moment.

» We can let go of judging past experiences and possible future outcomes.

» When we've made choices about where we want to go from here, we can have patience in the process of life.

» As we live each day, we can practice acceptance of whatever comes up.

» Day by day, we learn the balance necessary to move forward toward specific goals by setting priorities and letting go of attachments to specific outcomes, thoughts, or feelings.

» Finally, we can do all of this while living in the present moment, without expectation of some future goal or dream.

Dr. Matt often shares this story when discussing the power of planning as a part of this week's focus in our program:

I remember reading a self-help book when I was in my first year of medical school. It described the universe as a giant restaurant and the present moment as a time when you could place your order. The book recommended that you think clearly about what you wanted, and ask for specifics. Once that order was placed, there would be no chance to change your mind, so you needed to be sure that you placed your order correctly.

I gave my complete attention to the exercise, thinking about what was important to me—roles, abilities, relationships, accomplishments, and so on—and then placed my order, writing it down in a journal. I didn't revisit my order or make any changes on that piece of paper. Twenty-five years later, I went back to that journal, and every single part of that order had been filled—down to details like number of children and facilitating group work at a retreat center. The interesting thing is that when I made that list, I thought that if all of these requests came to fruition, I would be completely satisfied and perfectly content. Honest reflection revealed that I felt about the same way as when I made that list.

There was no magical field of happiness. Some of the requests had created joy and some had created suffering. Upon the realization that my order had been filled, I asked a friend what to do next. His reply: "Make a new list." But that did not sit well with me. Ultimately, I came to the realization that inhabiting all of these aspects of my life fully was the most important thing that I could do.

In understanding my dominant personality type (Enthusiast), I recognized that planning is one method that I habitually use to avoid being in the present moment. Realizing this, I've brought my focus to fully being in my life, instead of constantly striving and planning to get somewhere else. In addition, I am thankful that planning helped create a framework for that living. I'm very careful about what I ask for; this experience has clearly taught me that it is what I will receive.

Creating a personal mission statement

For this exercise, it's best to use your journal or some pen and paper to write down your thoughts. Each portion of the exercise builds on the next.

Bring your attention to the present moment by focusing on your breath. Aware that you are breathing in. Aware that you are breathing out.

- » Bring your focus to the following question: What do you most value in life? Write down your values.
- » Next bring your focus to the roles that you would like to play in life. Write them down.

» Now take a few minutes to reflect on what you value and roles that you would like to play in life. What would it look like if the roles aligned with your values? Line up your roles with the corresponding values. You can use the values more than once.

» Now, take some time to prioritize your matched roles and values. Make two categories: A and B. Under category A, place the most important matched role/value mix. Under category B, place the remaining role/values. (For an example, please see the Resource section on our Website at *sustainablewellnessonline.com*) How do your priorities, revealed in this exercise, match up with your actions?

» Now it's time to begin placing your order. Imagine that you're sitting in the restaurant of life and you're given a menu full of any possible roles and values that life has to offer. You can use your list to inform your order. Bring all of your creativity and attention to this process. When you place your order, imagine that you cannot change it. Imagine that whatever you order will be filled. The timing and places of fulfillment may vary, but a clearly placed order will be filled.

» Write down what you want your life to look like—the roles you want to play, accomplishments, ways of living—the more detailed, the better. Put this list somewhere safe. Once you have finished the list, resist the urge to change or tweak it.

» Now, look at your list and develop a daily statement of intention that is consistent with all aspects of the list coming into fruition. You can call this a personal mission statement.

This is all that is required. If it appeals to you, develop a list of goals and objectives that are consistent with parts of your order. You can choose to remind yourself of your personal mission by writing it down and posting it where you'll see it often. You could also say your mission statement daily as a part of your health practice.

This planning exercise is a way for you to personally experience the power of your intention. There is nothing magical or mysterious about it, and you can learn a great deal about yourself in the process.

Review

≫ We can bring our present-moment awareness to the past in order to better understand how where we have been influences where we are right now.

≫ Understanding can bring about gratitude and forgiveness, and these can provide inspiration for our life practice.

≫ Multiple participants in our life influence us on all levels of our being—mind, body, and spirit—and these influences are felt through multiple lenses—our personality, culture, and the natural world in which we live. We also have an impact on these areas outside of our personal self.

≫ We can bring our present-moment awareness to the future and develop a mission in life without getting lost in planning and missing the here and now.

Yoga Bits

≫ Share a story about yourself with a trusted friend or family member.

≫ Plant a tree that has the potential to last for a hundred years.

≫ In safe space, share something about yourself that you don't normally share in polite conversation.

≫ At the end of the day, think about things that you're thankful for from that day.

≫ Look for things during the day that surprise you, touch your heart, or inspire you. When you notice one of these, stop and take a single conscious breath in and out.

PART II
BEGINNING AGAIN: STEPS 4–8

Now that we've reached a turning point, let's review where this healing journey has taken us. In week 1, we began with the first step, cultivating awareness, as a foundation for all that we will do. In weeks 2 and 3, we've taken this ability to focus and turned inward, reflecting on who we are, where we have been, and where we want to go.

In the process, we've cultivated the ability to witness whatever comes up and to give space to thoughts, feelings, memories, and goals without trying to fix things. We've learned the value of cultivating the ability to stop, calm, rest, and heal. Whether the plan we created lasts 30 years or 30 days, we've developed a vision for life based on our values, and we've committed to looking at that life with mercy and awareness. We've emptied our cup and entered the world of healing.

This process allows us to participate in life as we never have before by seeing all things with new eyes. It encourages us to let go of assumptions and to embrace choices in the present moment. Neuroscientists believe that 90 percent of our decision-making is based on subconscious, knee-jerk reactions. The brain quickly becomes hardwired to react in the ways it has reacted before. Awareness and mindful practice help us tame this natural tendency. In time, automatic reactions give way to considered responses.

As we move into this next phase together, it's helpful to think of the mind as a garden planted with many dormant seeds. Some of these seeds are found in everyone, as a consequence of being human. Some are planted out of habit and some by choice. Individually, we may have more or less of any particular seed based on personality type, genetic heritage, where we live, and so on. Our life experience, both internal and external, tends to water certain seeds. When a seed is watered it's nourished, and it finds the strength to burst through the soil. Eventually, it may sprout, grow, and yield fruit. The fruit that comes from each seed is unique, and is a direct result of the nature of the seed. Some of the fruit will be bitter, and some will be sweet. When the seed of anger is watered in our mind's garden, the resulting fruit will taste far different from fruit grown from the seed of gratitude.

The mind's hardwired habit energy works in fast motion, and the force of habit speeds up our knee-jerk reactions. When a seed is watered, it grows, blooms, and produces fruit almost instantaneously if it's set strongly in the soil. Its strength is in proportion to its nourishment and roots. If we constantly water a particular seed, through our own actions or by exposure to other's actions, it will quickly produce a more potent fruit. If we are very attached or averse to a particular seed, the energy of this attachment or aversion will nourish it.

In this phase of our journey, we enter active areas of our lives and what we think of as "doing." We eat (nutrition). We move (physical activity). We think and feel (mind-body stress management). We find meaning (spirituality).

These activities can easily begin to define us. Despite the difficulty of letting go of old worries and releasing future expectations, the greatest challenge may be right here in the present moment as we eat, move, think, feel, and find meaning, all while our seeds are watered. Practice can prepare us to notice stimuli when they occur and can inform our choices. But the real fruit of practice—of life—comes down to our actions.

Feels like a lot of pressure, doesn't it? Now add a world of infinite choices and possibilities! We're overwhelmed by diets, exercise programs, stress-reduction techniques, religions, and spiritual practices—all of them numbering in the hundreds and all of them more accessible through the ever-present media. *Have an eating disorder? Overweight? Obese? Stressed out? Squishy abs? Feeling lost? We have an app for that.*

There may be nothing inherently wrong with these potential programs or solutions. On the contrary, some of these tools can help keep our lives in balance and promote health and wellness. The problem comes when we get so attached to the tool itself that it becomes more important than our balance. When that happens, the process is destined to fail. When we become more focused on the tool than the original intention, it's only a matter of time before the approach becomes unsustainable. We fall off the wagon, resume old patterns, and water the same seeds of habit.

Sound familiar? So how do we begin again?

Healing with an integrative focus

We begin again by looking at all aspects of what we do with mercy and awareness, as they involve all levels of our being and experience in the process of life. We follow this practice in a safe space—one that holds in confidence whatever comes up without trying to fix it, preferably sharing our individual processes among people with similar life experience. Through this practice, our lives are transformed. We can integrate specific tools into our life practice in a way that serves us, rather than subjecting ourselves to the tool or regimen.

Through moment-by-moment awareness, we begin to observe which seeds are watered as it happens. This isn't possible for a mind filled with the continuous background noise of projects, desires, worries, thoughts, and feelings. When we are mindful, however, it's possible to see whatever comes up in the present moment. That awareness creates a space where we're able to choose how we respond to internal experience and external events.

There's a reason that the three-legged stool sits on the ground of awareness. Without it, balance is not possible. It would be like sitting on the stool while it floats weightless in outer space. With awareness, we become grounded and connected to our being. As we move forward, it's important to remember that although it's possible to overdo any facet or activity of life, it's nearly impossible to over-*be*. We will always begin with the practice of cultivating awareness because it's primary and foundational. When you find yourself floundering, feeling out of balance, or not sure where to turn, remember: Stop. Calm. Rest. Heal.

The three legs of the stool as an integrative process

For the remaining five chapters, we'll look at all three legs of the stool from the same integrative perspective that we used for the life review. We'll look through the filters of experience—the lenses of self, culture, and the natural world. We'll do this in a systematic way, beginning with the big-picture perspectives and progressively narrowing down to how each area affects us. Imagine starting at 50,000 feet viewing the entire landscape and finishing with your feet planted firmly on the ground, looking at the tiniest of details calmly.

Let's continue on our journey with steps 4 through 8.

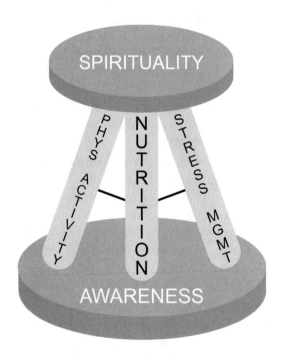

STEP 4:
NUTRITION

Preach not to others what they should eat, but eat as becomes you, and be silent.
—Epictetus, AD 55–135

*Y*ou are what you eat—and there are a lot of different foods. It's possible to cultivate a relationship with food that nourishes the mind and spirit as well as the body. We can begin to gauge our measure of fulfillment as well as our fullness. Too many dietary changes made at once can be stressful and difficult to sustain. Remember: New habits take time to develop. We will discuss building them with slow and consistent adjustments to diet and how and where we eat.

The roots of our many hungers can only be understood when patterns of consumption are recognized with patience and awareness. Be gentle and forgive yourself when you make less-than-perfect choices. Smile and begin again. The healing nourishment of self-acceptance is a powerful tool. This isn't an all-or-nothing proposition, but a new way of seeing the habits and tendencies developed throughout a lifetime.

Create a consumption diary to monitor your effort and progress. (You'll find an example of a consumption diary in the Resources section at *sustainablewellnessonline.com*) Gradually, new preferences will emerge, choice by choice and bite by bite. Our nutrition Yoga Bits can help keep the process practical and sustainable in the midst of your day.

Nourishment: All that feeds us

We need many kinds of nourishment to balance our mind, body, and spirit. Just as the body hungers for certain nutrients in order to function and thrive, the mind and heart also hunger for emotional and spiritual nourishment. Satisfying these many needs is a continuous and lifelong pursuit.

Nutrition is the "energy in" side of the equation that balances our life practice. When we consume anything, we take in its quality and absorb its effects. It works like the drops of food coloring that dissolve in the water supporting the white flower, slowly transforming its color. We may not notice immediate changes, but they'll occur in time as the qualities of what we consume affect our expression of life. Let's bring our focus and awareness to all that nourishes us using the same integrative framework we used for the life review. What we consume affects, and is affected by, much more than just our individual self. This integrative view affords us a comprehensive perspective that broadens the scope of our possible choices.

At times, we'll be faced with questions for which there are no clear-cut answers. The precautionary principle can be very helpful in making decisions about processes in which the effects are unknown or unclear. This principle states that if we don't know the definitive answer, and there is significant potential for harm based on what we do know, it's best to proceed with caution and avoid potential harm. This "first do no harm" approach can help guide our choices and provide a useful framework when we're not sure which way to turn.

When most people think about nutrition and nourishment, they think about edible food. This chapter will focus mainly on nutrition from this angle while still recognizing that everything we're exposed to feeds us in some way and at some level. Our days are organized around meal times, and what we eat highlights our social activities and celebrations. Food preparations are unique to cultures and regions, and traditions and eating habits follow us through generations. It seems that our relationship with food is one of life's most complex. While choice and quantity of food may overwhelm some of us, a growing number people find it a scant resource. At extremes, obesity destroys some lives while starvation ravages others.

This chapter will discuss ways to expand our perspective and explore how changes in what we consume affect our community, region, nation, and Earth itself. This may seem a little daunting at first, but we'll help guide you through the process. Our integrative review will include questions about how you approach life in each category. Many of these questions are open-ended, and your answers can change throughout a lifetime. They are useful guides as we approach our food and consumption choices with greater awareness, and they can help you sustain healthy consumption patterns. If you notice major areas of concern, try to address these with small interventions to balance out the situation. For example, if you decide that eating red meat reduces the availability of resources for other people on the planet, you could try substituting it with more plant-based food options. Let's begin.

Nutrition and all participants

There are only so many resources available on our planet, and our consumption patterns affect others in tangible ways. We can make more informed choices when we invite a broader perspective on consumption that includes our family and grows to include our community, society, country, and planet. As you go through the remainder of our integrative review, keep the following questions in mind.

Questions to ponder:

» When we apply awareness to what we consume, we may notice the potential for harm or good that any food or beverage offers. Can we use the precautionary principle as a guide to our consumption? What do we currently consume that has the potential for harm? Why do we still choose to ingest it?

» How important is it for your consumption to have a neutral or positive effect on every being living on the earth? Is this even possible?

» How important is it that your consumption has a positive effect on your country, community, and family? Are there different levels of importance for each? Why?

≫ How can you change your consumption habits to have a positive effect on others in the process? The work of sustainable wellness relies on making continuous, small adjustments over time based on your current needs for balance. Because our balance can affect the balance of others, it's important to choose carefully.

≫ How do your consumption habits have a negative effect on others, such as people living in another part of the world? Is there some small step that you can make to address this imbalance?

Nutrition and the natural world

In this section, we'll first discuss how our food choices impact the natural world. We'll then cover how our sense of sight can guide us to miraculous foods and optimal nutrition. Because supplements are sometimes necessary (due to farming practices and their impact on the natural world), a discussion is also included with references to resources.

The cycle of all life

The food that we eat reaches our table after a long journey. That journey begins in the natural world, including the soil, clouds, rain, air, and sunshine. What ends up on our plate is made from all of these components. If any one of these resources were removed, the end product would no longer exist. The natural world actually becomes our food. Our food goes through a long chain of processing and handling by farmers, laborers, transporters, grocers, and cooks. If we take out any link from that chain, our food wouldn't reach our table. We can appreciate that the efforts of many people are necessary in order to feed just one. When we eat the food in front of us, we smell, taste, chew, digest, and then excrete what isn't needed. The food literally becomes our body, and what we don't use returns to the earth. The cycle begins again.

In the Introduction, we presented geometry's transitive property. If A = B and B = C, then A = C. If the natural world equals our food, and our food equals our body, then our body equals the natural world. When we eat, we consume the sunshine, the clouds, and the soil, and we also digest food and recycle waste back to the earth. How does this knowledge affect how we choose to eat? As we maintain balance in our life and body, how do we ensure balance in the natural world?

Put simply, there's a link between what we choose to eat and balance in the natural world. For example, the production of beef uses significantly greater resources to grow and deliver than producing plants with the same nutritional benefit. Production of beef requires greater input from the natural world—more water, land, and food to feed the cows, and recycling of wastes—than what's required for the production of plants. Animal farming is more taxing on nature and less sustainable than plant farming. We can feed more people in a healthy and sustainable way by eating a diet that is focused on whole foods, mostly plants.

Organic food

The nutrients in our food come from the soil, and certain types of plants contain specific types of nutrients. If the same plants are placed in the same soil over and over, eventually they'll stop growing because all of the essential nutrients will have been leached from the soil. Nutrient depletion in both soil and plants is a consequence of major farm operations that reuse the same piece of land and exhaust its resources. The widespread use of pesticides and fertilizers is necessary to make the large-scale production of any food source more practical and economically viable. Most scientists say that large-scale production has a potentially harmful impact on living beings.

Organic foods are raised without inorganic chemical pesticides or fertilizers, and when organic farmers carefully recycle organic waste and rotate crops, the soil is replenished. One benefit of organic fruits and vegetables over non-organic foods is that the organic plants must fight harder to survive and thrive. In order to do this, they develop phytonutrients as defenses all on their own, without the support of processed chemicals. One theory is that as they develop greater quantities of these nutrients, they deliver higher nutritional value when consumed.

Organic food production is more expensive per piece of food than large-scale, chemical-based industrial operations because it costs more money to replenish soil with organic fertilizer and keep plants healthy with proper watering and pest removal. For many, it may not be financially practical to eat only organic. If we do choose to eat more organic foods, how can we prioritize our choices and stay within a budget? The United States Department of Agriculture (USDA) studied which foods are more likely to have high levels of pesticide residue. This investigation led to the Dirty Dozen and the Clean 15 lists.[1] When possible, it's best to eat organic forms of the foods that appear on the Dirty Dozen list.

Dirty Dozen (buy these organic)

- Apples
- Strawberries
- Celery
- Peaches
- Spinach
- Imported nectarines
- Imported grapes
- Sweet bell peppers
- Potatoes
- Domestic blueberries
- Lettuce
- Kale/collard greens

Clean 15 (lowest in pesticides)

- Onions
- Sweet corn
- Pineapples
- Avocado
- Asparagus
- Sweet peas
- Mangoes
- Eggplant
- Domestic cantaloupe
- Kiwi
- Cabbage
- Watermelon
- Sweet potatoes
- Grapefruit
- Mushrooms

You can write or print these lists on a small card to keep with you while shopping. Generally speaking, foods with higher pesticide exposure have a thinner outer skin or protective layer, whereas those with a thicker outer skin are more naturally hardy and require fewer pesticides to grow.

Supplements, colors, or both?

Ideally, all of the vitamins and minerals needed to support optimal health would be present in a diet that includes a variety of vegetables and fruits. One good way to help the body get what it needs is to eat a diet that has the entire spectrum of colors in it. Different nutrients have different chemical structures and produce different colors. Simply including a rainbow of colors on your plate can help ensure that you're getting the proper spectrum of vitamins and minerals. Our color spectrum table can be helpful in choosing a rainbow palette of foods. (See Table 4–1).

FOOD COLOR CHART	
RED	Beets, cherries, cranberries, radishes, raspberries, red apples, red grapes, red peppers, strawberries, tomatoes, watermelons
GREEN	Asparagus, arugula, avocados, broccoli, Brussels sprouts, celery, cucumbers, green apples, green beans, green grapes, green peppers, kiwis, leafy greens, lettuce, limes, okra, peas, spinach, zucchini
YELLOW/ ORANGE	Apricots, butternut squash, cantaloupes, carrots, grapefruits, lemons, mangoes, oranges, peaches, pineapples, pumpkins, sweet potatoes, yellow apples, yellow tomatoes
BLUE/PURPLE	Blackberries, blueberries, dried plums, eggplants, grapes, purple cabbage, purple peppers, raisins
WHITE	Bananas, cauliflower, garlic, ginger, mushrooms, onions, turnips, white corns, white nectarines

Table 4–1: Food Color Chart

How does soil depletion impact vitamin and mineral absorption in humans? What about other nutrients that may not be present even in a whole-food, plant-based diet? Are vitamin and mineral supplements necessary? These are controversial issues, and there's no right or wrong answer. For individuals with high toxin loads from smoking, certain chemically synthesized supplements, such as beta-carotene, can actually increase cancer risk. On the other hand, broad-spectrum supplementation with compounds that closely mimic nutrients found in foods may be helpful in disease prevention. It's important to recognize that supplements do not provide everything we need, and they can't replace a whole-food, plant-based diet. The data on this is clear. You just can't overwhelm your body with ingestible poisons like tobacco, alcohol, charred red meat, processed foods, and refined sugar, and hope that supplements will fix everything. However, given the fact that it's difficult to obtain all that we need from our foods as they are today, there may be a role for both foundational and targeted supplements.

There are several supplements that address these issues. It makes sense to include a good multivitamin, omega-3 fatty acids, calcium, and vitamin D3. The supplement page in the Resources section on our Website suggests where you can find good quality products in the appropriate amounts. Probiotics are also reasonable additions. They are beneficial bacteria that reside in the gut and help break down food so the proper nutrients can be digested. For many of the same reasons that vitamins and minerals have been depleted from soil, these beneficial bacteria have also been depleted. Through the process of natural fermentation, yogurt and sauerkraut contain many of these beneficial organisms. It's reasonable to add fermented foods to your diet, or take a probiotic supplement. Several options for these supplements are listed in the Resources section on our Website. A good Website that provides an integrative, individualized assessment and recommendations for supplementation is *www.drweilvitaminadvisor.com*.

If you follow a whole-food, plant-based diet, there are certain vitamins that you'll need to take as supplements—specifically, vitamin B12. Food sources of B12 generally come from the animal world, mainly dairy and eggs, though some vegetarian foods are fortified with B12. If you have recently become a vegetarian, it can take from three to 20 years to deplete B12 stores already built up in your body. This vitamin is an essential part of maintaining a healthy nervous system and also helps in creating new blood cells and DNA. B12 deficiencies can result in anemia and nervous system disorders. A decent multivitamin should contain about 2mcg of B12, or Cyanocobalamin, in order to provide the recommended daily allowance.

Certainly, what we choose to consume and how we choose to consume it directly affects the natural world. We can learn to use only what is necessary and prevent waste and harm to the environment. In so doing, we'll ultimately prevent harm to ourselves.

Nutrition and our culture

Picture the following scene: It's a day in November and an entire family is gathered around a table that's overflowing with food. A huge meal is consumed, with enough food to feed that same family for many days. Looking at that meal from a typical American perspective, it's a happy Thanksgiving. Viewed from another cultural perspective or upbringing, it may seem completely different.

Think about what your culture tells you about what you need in order to be nourished. Does your culture focus on consumption as a means to an end? Are certain foods encouraged? Are others disdained? Are there certain rituals that surround eating food or taking in nourishment? Think about how your understanding of your cultural tendencies can affect your daily practices. Do you view food as a reward or celebration? If so, how does this affect your consumption?

Nutrition and the lens of self

Along with family traditions and culture, our individual personalities shape how we nourish ourselves. Use the following questions to consider how your dominant personality type influences your food choices.

Questions to ponder:

» Do you take in a broad selection, or only the foods you like?

» Do you eat large amounts at one time or sparingly throughout the day?

» Do you consider why you eat certain foods and avoid others?

» How does your personality type's basic fear and desire affect your consumption patterns?

» How do you eat when you feel balanced and healthy compared to when you feel out of balance?

» How does your ego fixation relate to how you eat?

Our basic fear and basic desire can influence our approach to what and how much we consume. As you bring your focused awareness to these questions it will allow you to recognize patterns that either support or inhibit your balance.

Nutrition and the mind

Food is experienced in the mind as well as the mouth. Along with nutrients, we're fed by the color, smell, texture, and flavor of foods. Unfortunately, the speed of our multitasking world gives us little opportunity to enjoy the simple pleasures of eating. Often, we're too distracted by a television or computer screen to appreciate what's on the plate in front of us—if we even use a plate. We wolf down fast foods on the run and use instant foods to save even more time. We eat mindlessly, with little thought to what we ingest and how it affects body, mind, and spirit.

Take the time to consider how food makes you feel and what's on your mind when you eat. Think about how taking in new energy makes you feel, and how you know when to stop eating. Is it easy for you to tell when you have reached the satiety level, or is it a difficult process? Do you often eat meals without paying any attention to the food in front of you?

Mindful eating is a helpful tool in understanding the answers to some of these questions. When we eat mindfully, we stop and bring our calm focus to the food that is directly in front of us. We're aware of its appeal and how we came to consume it. As we begin to eat, we keep our focus on the entire process at hand, rather than getting lost in some other thought or task.

Let the following exercise guide you through a mindful eating experience.

Exercise: Mindful eating

What you will need:

≫ About 10 minutes

≫ A piece of one of your favorite foods that you can easily hold in your hand

≫ A quiet place

Find a comfortable position, preferably with your feet flat on the floor and sitting down straight with awareness. Focus on your breath as it makes your belly rise and fall. Place your hand on your belly and observe how your hand rises and falls with each breath. Take a minute and close your eyes. Allow your awareness to ride the wave of your breath.

Now bring your focus to the piece of your favorite food. Pick it up and look closely at it, as though you had never seen anything like it before. Where did it come from? Are there any clues as to its origins? Imagine all that occurred to bring this piece of food you're holding in your hand—its growth, nurturing, handling, and transport. Examine all of its characteristics: colors, contours, and patterns.

If you find your mind wandering, bring your focus back to the breath and then back to the piece of food. Next, explore the mass of the food. Feel its contours with your fingers. Notice its weight as you lift it up and down in the palm of your hand. Now bring it to your nose and smell it. Inhale and exhale the aroma of this piece of food. Does it smell different from one nostril to the other? Does the smell bring up any memories or thoughts? If so, gently and firmly bring your focus back to the food itself.

Now open your mouth and place it on your tongue. Feel its weight in your mouth. Roll it around in your mouth a little. Notice any sensations. Does it feel different in your mouth than in your hand? Have you started salivating? Do you have an urge to chew and swallow it? Is there any taste before chewing? What does it feel like to anticipate chewing and swallowing the piece of food?

Now, close your eyes and slowly begin to chew the food and notice all of the sensations you experience: the taste, your body's response to chewing in the form of saliva, the urge to swallow, and so on. Slowly chew the food. Notice how the feel of this piece of food has changed. Notice the taste and how your body reacts.

Now begin to swallow. As you swallow, notice how this happens. Focus on how the food goes down the esophagus and eventually ends up in the stomach. See if you can feel this entire process. After some time, give thanks for this piece of food and the nourishment that it will provide you. Notice how it feels to have eaten it. Are you more satisfied than you would expect from this small amount?

When you are ready, slowly open your eyes, bring your focus back to your breath, and back to your body in the chair, then back to the surroundings in the room.

Take a few moments afterward to answer the following questions:

1. What was this experience like for you?
2. How is mindful eating different from how you usually eat?
3. How is it the same?
4. How can you build some of this practice into your daily eating habits?
5. How do you think that it might be helpful?
6. Are there barriers to bringing this practice into your daily life?

To apply this practice to your daily life, take one conscious breath before beginning to eat or drink anything. Then bring your focus and attention to what you consume.

Why do we eat?

Nutrition has become one of the most emotion-laden subjects in our world today. Some have too much food and some have too little. There are comfort foods, guilty pleasures, yo-yo dieting, and much more. Take some time to recognize and name how you may be caught up in some of these habits and patterns surrounding food and consumption. For example, if you find yourself eating a great deal after coming home from a busy day at work, focus and awareness may help you realize that you are eating to relax or find comfort. You can identify and name this process "eating to manage stress." By naming the situation, you take away a great deal of its power. Naming introduces a little space to make a conscious choice and manage your stress differently. Some options might be going for a walk or mindfully drinking a cup of relaxing tea, such as chamomile, which also soothes the stomach.

This is an excellent area to practice patience and non-judgment. An extra piece of chocolate doesn't have to be consumed with a side of guilt! When consumed mindfully and freely, an occasional small treat might be enough to satisfy. We can consciously choose to eat smaller portions of treats and pick ones that have higher nutritional value. Rather than drinking a chocolate milk shake, we can choose a more full-flavored and nutritious piece of dark chocolate. It's also a good idea to consider feeding our body throughout the day, rather than consuming only two or three large meals. Five or six small meals can limit the overeating that often happens with larger meals. It can also help prevent feeling tired as our body works to digest large amounts of food eaten all at once.

Nutrition and the body

Physical hunger is one of the very first sensations we experience as newborns and one of the last to fade as we approach old age and death. It can be a very powerful motivator. Physical hunger directly addresses our basic survival needs. For most of you reading this book, these needs are met. We are looking for what meets them in the most balanced way possible. What is the best nutritional plan for physical health?

There is much to address in order to bring full understanding to this topic. Certainly, there are no fixed solutions that are correct for everyone. Important considerations include: the type of diet that is best for an individual, when an individual should eat to maximize physical health, and how much an individual should eat. The key word here is *individual.* Modern science can reduce the body's nutritional requirements to the molecular level, and food is often considered the fuel that powers the human machine. However, the entire person needs to be taken into account, not just nutritional science.

Many diet plans focus entirely on weight loss. In this case, a diet is considered something that one goes on and then goes off. By definition, this is not a sustainable approach. There are also diets that are associated with specific cultures; the Mediterranean Diet and the Standard American Diet are two examples. Here, the word *diet* is more associated with the sustained general practices of a group than with a weight-loss or goal-oriented plan. Our approach will be to focus on diet as a daily part of your life.

What does your body need in order to function optimally? There are several considerations that address this question:

» Your body needs to have a certain number of calories available for consumption in order to meet the demands of living, whatever that may be for you. The caloric needs of an elite athlete in training are definitely different than those of a sedentary office worker. The Resources section on our Website lists a way to figure out your daily calorie needs.

» Your body needs food to be properly digested and moved through the gastrointestinal system, ending with appropriate excretion of what is not needed. In that digestion process, you need a mix of carbohydrates, fats, fiber, and proteins in order to fill the demand for tissue use and repair. The optimal mix will vary for individuals, but a range includes the following:

» Carbohydrates: 45–65% of calories

» Protein: 10–35% of calories

» Fat: 20–35% of calories

» Fiber: 22–34 grams per day

» You require a broad array of vitamins, minerals, and enzymes in order to keep all of your physical processes functioning smoothly. The majority of these are provided by a whole-food, plant-based diet. The Resources section at *sustainablewellnessonline.com* lists foundational supplement recommendations.

» You require clean water for every cell in the body to function properly. Water makes up 60 percent of your body weight and is constantly used and lost in normal activity. Generally speaking, you should drink about 80 ounces of clean, purified water every day. Reverse osmosis is the best method to remove impurities from properly sanitized tap water.

When you take in more calories than you put out in energetic effort, the excess calories are stored for future use. Eventually, the stored calories are converted into fat. Generally, there are health consequences when you take in too much or too little carbohydrates, fats, protein, fiber, vitamins, minerals, or water. Likewise, there are consequences for consuming unhealthy substances, such as charred red meat cooked with high heat. What other foods place your body in a state of imbalance?

Over time, science has developed new chemically synthesized compounds that have the same taste and feel of actual food products, and they also have distinct advantages for the marketplace. Many of these new chemicals give us the ability to process whole foods so they have a greater shelf life. They also take advantage of abundantly available resources, such as corn. Most of us are familiar with the two most common examples: trans fatty acids, which are used in place of natural fats that spoil quickly, and high-fructose corn syrup, which is derived from overly abundant corn and used as a sweetener.

You can try an interesting experiment to experience firsthand the difference between natural foods that have evolved in time and been around for eons, and foods that have been processed with the help of synthetic substances and modern manufacturing. Place a commercially available snack cake and an apple in the trunk of your car. Put the apple in a plastic bag and keep the snack cake in its wrapper. Leave them in there for a month. After one month, the apple will have rotted away to nearly nothing. The snack cake will still be ready to eat (and will taste pretty good!).

So why not eat only scientifically derived miracle foods that last forever? Well, when humans ingest processed foods containing chemically synthesized compounds, multiple well-documented problems can occur. Much of our society's problem with obesity and chronic disease focuses on the effects of high-fructose corn syrup and trans fatty acids, though there are many other types of compounds around. Take a look at a commercial box of cookies or a bag of chips. Go down to the ingredients section and see how many words you find that aren't food. You'll be able to spot these because they're difficult to pronounce. These are either chemicals derived from food or preservatives to keep the food-derived elements from spoiling on the shelf. How exactly do these foreign products affect the body?

Inflammation and diet

Eating processed foods creates inflammation in the body. Inflammation sets the stage for chronic health problems such as heart disease, arthritis, diabetes, and cancer. The chemically synthesized compounds found in processed foods aren't digested like the compounds found in natural foods that have been around for hundreds of years. Our bodies digest and store them differently, and this produces specific chemical reactions. These reactions cause internal inflammation. And although some level of inflammation is necessary for the body to function, massive uncontrolled levels damage the whole system.

Imagine that the body is like a house. Every house needs a place to cook food. Under normal circumstances, this is limited to the kitchen stove. An optimally functioning house has this resource confined and controlled in a single area, with multiple safeguards surrounding the area of heat generation. An optimally functioning body is the same. If a house had kitchen stoves in every room, and no safeguards around to keep the heating areas under control, the excess heat might burn the whole house down. If it did catch fire, it would be hard to locate the source and extinguish the flames. A body that is ravaged by system-wide inflammation is the same. In a balanced approach to sustainable wellness, specific organs provide safe levels of inflammation and function where and when they're needed. The stomach secretes acid and enzymes to help digest and process food, and this produces a controlled inflammatory chemical reaction.

So what else causes inflammation on a body-wide basis? We know that carrying around too much weight, or unused stored calories, can cause inflammation in a variety of ways. One way to gauge your risk for inflammation from excess body weight is to calculate your Body Mass Index (BMI). This index is a ratio of your weight to your height (see the Website Resources section.) If you are on the extremes of this scale—in either the very low, malnourished category, or the very high, obese category—then you may be at higher risk for health problems related to inflammation. The BMI is not a perfect indicator of excess body weight from fat and should be used only as a guide along with many other measures of your health. For example, it's also important to know your waist circumference. Women with a waist circumference greater than 35 inches, and men with a waist circumference of greater than 40 inches, may be at higher risk for illness.

There are some other characteristics of food that can affect inflammation. The glycemic index is a measure of how quickly a particular food is converted into the usable fuel of blood glucose. If a food is digested very quickly into sugar, it has a high glycemic index, and if it is digested very slowly, it has a low glycemic index. Basically, foods that the body works hard to digest into sugar molecules have a lower glycemic index, because the body actually expends energy to break them apart. Foods that quickly go to blood sugar indirectly create inflammation in many areas by multiple mechanisms, including excessive hormone release to handle the sugar surge.

Another important consideration is the glycemic load. The glycemic load is the amount of carbohydrate that is in a food adjusted for how quickly it turns into blood sugar. It's important to know how easily the body turns food into sugar, as well as the quantity or carbohydrate grams per serving. Your blood sugar rises and falls when you consume a food, and this depends on how quickly it's converted to sugar in the body, as well as the quantity of calories per serving.

Generally whole foods have a lower glycemic index and load than those that have been processed and manufactured into more convenient storage and delivery systems. Orange juice has a glycemic index of 46 and a glycemic load of 12, and a whole orange has a glycemic index of 33–48 and a glycemic load of 3–6. A single serving of orange juice raises blood sugar more in a shorter period of time than a single orange does due to increased calories. Please see the Website *www.glycemicindex.com* for a thorough list of ratings for many foods. There may be several listings for the same food. Use the listing for comparisons between foods and try to stick with whole, unprocessed foods that have a lower glycemic load. Eat foods closest to their natural form.

Certain foods are directly anti-inflammatory and some are directly pro-inflammatory. Many years ago, it was recognized that Eskimos who ate large quantities of wild-caught salmon rich in omega-3 fats rarely developed heart disease. Omega-3 fatty acids found in walnuts, flax seed, and cold-water fish (like salmon) are anti-inflammatory, whereas chemically manufactured trans fatty acids found in most processed foods are pro-inflammatory. Certain spices, like ginger and turmeric, have significant anti-inflammatory characteristics. An anti-inflammatory diet includes a focus on these directly beneficial foods, using supplements where needed (see the Website Resources section), while limiting directly pro-inflammatory substances.

Noticing whole foods

So what types of whole foods are best to eat and which are best to avoid if our goal is to decrease inflammation overall? When looking at food, let's first define what the word *food* means. For our purposes, food is something we consume that offers nutritional value and has not been substantially altered from its original state. A grain of wheat, a kernel of corn, and an apple are entirely different from their highly processed versions used to create a sugar-laden, nutritionally fortified children's breakfast cereal. The whole grain, kernel, and fruit are foods. The cereal is a processed food product (PFP).

We'd like to introduce a creative test to differentiate food from a PFP: *The Noticing Whole Food Time Machine*. Imagine that you own a time machine and can go back in time to visit your ancestors living a hundred years ago. Take whatever food you're interested in into that time machine, and show it to your distant relative. If they've never seen it, heard of it, smelled it, or tasted it, and it's not available to them anywhere on the planet, then it's probably a PFP and not a food.

PFPs cause inflammation many times greater than most whole foods. When trying to determine whether a specific product will promote health and help keep inflammation at healthy levels, first ask yourself: Is this a whole food or a PFP? If it's a PFP, limit your use in order to reduce inflammation.

A second consideration is more controversial and just as important. If what you're interested in is a whole food, is it from an animal or a plant? Animal-based foods tend to be more pro-inflammatory than plant-based foods. From the standpoint of inflammation, it's healthier to eat plants than animals. There's a great deal of scientific literature to support this statement, despite previous recommendations that dairy and meat products be a major part of a healthy diet. The best information available concerning this comes from researcher Colin Campbell and is well documented in his book, *The China Study*.[2] Basically, Campbell showed that animal-based diets cause greater risk of chronic disease development than plant-based diets. This conclusion was based on a 20-year study that looked at death rates from 48 forms of cancer and other chronic diseases from 65 counties in China. Each of these individual counties contained a stable population of individuals who were genetically similar, with shared lifestyle and dietary habits. Counties with high consumption of animal products had higher rates of death from cancer and chronic disease.

What to eat

A whole-food, plant-based diet is the optimal diet to follow in order to keep inflammation at healthy levels. You don't have to eat only plant-based products (though that may be advised for some individuals), but it's best to get at least 80 percent of your nutrition from plants. What are whole parts of plants? Any of the foods listed in Table 4–1 are certainly included. We can eat the fruit, nuts, stem, leaves, and plant roots in their whole form in order to take in the highest nutrient and fiber level, and the best glycemic load. Often when these whole parts are processed, nutrients and fiber are lost. This makes the food less healthy and may turn it into a PFP that our distant relative wouldn't recognize.

Consume fresh grains, vegetables, and fruits as the foundation of your diet. It's a common misconception that plant foods don't contain enough protein and, therefore, we must consume animal products. See *www .sustainablewellnessonline.com* for whole plant-based foods that contain significant amounts of protein. If you decide to eat animal protein, choose a part from the whole animal that hasn't been processed into a meat product. Ideally, meat would come from animals raised in a natural environment that haven't been fed toxic compounds or injected with antibiotics and growth hormones. Organic, free-range animal products raised on farms that operate like those a hundred years ago are best. If you brought your distant relatives to a modern commercial dairy or cattle operation, they'd think they were visiting an alien world. Processed animal products are just as dangerous as processed plant products.

There are certain foods that you should eat and some that you should avoid. We recommend avoiding all PFPs, as much as possible. We also recommend avoiding charred meats and moldy grain foods, such as moldy bread products that have passed their recommended date for consumption and have visible mold growing on the surface. When eating meat, choose lean products and cook them thoroughly, at a low temperature for a long time (low and slow).

From a beverage standpoint, water has generally become a PFP. Go ahead and take some tap water back in your time machine and ask your relatives for yourself. They very likely wouldn't recognize the smell or taste of our processed water. We can use the precautionary principle as a guide and recommend that you drink clean water, purified through reverse osmosis to remove all of the chemicals that aren't filtered out normally, such as the chemicals we use to clean the water. Avoid all other liquid PFPs. This includes sodas and most juices. Remember the time-machine test if you are unsure. Green tea is an outstanding beverage choice with multiple well-documented health benefits. (See "How to brew a great cup of green tea" at *www.sustainablewellnessonline.com*.)

When you eat is also important. It's a good idea to avoid eating large amounts of food at any one sitting because it affects digestion, blood sugar, and inflammation levels. An optimal schedule is eating at least five times per day, including breakfast, a midmorning snack, lunch, a midafternoon snack, dinner, and an optional post-dinner snack.

You can figure out how many calories you need by looking at the chart in the Resources section. Limit the quantity of foods you consume that have a high caloric density, such as nuts. A few of these can carry quite a caloric punch. There's a great old saying about food: "Eat breakfast like a king, lunch like a prince, and dinner like a pauper." Avoid eating large amounts at bedtime so that your body, including your digestive system, has time to rest.

Certain compounds deserve special mention. Avoid tobacco products (need we say more?). Avoid significant amounts of alcohol. Most would consider a significant amount more than one alcoholic beverage per day. Whereas there may be some health benefit to a daily glass of red wine, this same health benefit comes from eating whole grapes that contain the same beneficial nutrients, including resveratrol. From a cancer-prevention standpoint, there is no safe daily amount of alcohol.

We've created some sample menus in the Resources section on our Website, a list of some superfoods, and some recipes for healthy smoothies to start off the day. Healthy smoothies are a practical and tasty way to get in clean protein and multiple servings of fruits and vegetables. The protein can come from a clean animal source such as whey, or from a plant source such as soy, rice, or hemp. Whey protein is a clean-burning fuel derived from dairy milk that provides health benefits, whereas casein is a pro-inflammatory milk protein that can lead to health problems.

When making changes in your diet, it's good to begin with a goal in mind. If we've convinced you of the value of a whole-food, plant-based diet, start with some minor adjustments and take a small step. You might begin with a healthy smoothie in the morning, substituting whole, plant foods for fast foods during the day, taking appropriate foundational supplements, eating more often to avoid overeating, decreasing intake of processed sugary foods, or drinking clean filtered water. You can pick any of these to start, and add a new change every week until your diet looks as close to your goal as possible.

Nutrition and the spirit

Jesus of Nazareth is arguably one of the greatest teachers who ever walked the planet. The night before he knew he was to be arrested and put to death, he gathered all of his students. He taught them a specific exercise, and a very important one given the setting. He broke bread and said that the bread was his body. He drank wine and said that the wine was his blood. He asked that his students practice this exercise. The food and drink that we consume literally becomes our body and blood. This is a very deep practice of mindful eating that links us to the natural world and to each other.

From a spiritual perspective, how does what we consume help us to align with our final and highest concern? How does it hinder us? How can we make the way we consume into a spiritual practice?

Exploration: A consumption diary

The following exercise is a good way to bring awareness to all you consume. First, think about what nourishes you on all levels. Next, think about yesterday. Jot down everything you consumed from the moment you woke up until you went to sleep. Now begin with a new day and write down everything you consume, as you consume it. Include what, when, where, how much, and why. Then compare the two days. Are there any differences or similarities? This exploration may reveal what happens when we bring our focus and present-moment awareness to what we're eating. Keep this consumption diary as a part of your daily practice journal, especially whenever you make a change in your eating habits. It's a helpful way to gauge any changes as time goes on. (See *www .sustainablewellnessonline.com* for an example of a consumption diary.)

Practice: Growing your own food

Pick a spot where you can grow some of your own food. It can be as small and simple as a single flowerpot. It might be an herb or a tomato plant. Mindfully plant seeds or place a whole plant in the soil, and make sure that it has adequate nutrients and water to survive. You may want to say a brief prayer whenever you plant something new, asking for its health and growth. Each time you tend to your garden, you might follow this brief focusing exercise.

As I breathe in, I tend to my garden,
As I breathe out, I am thankful.
Tending to my garden,
Thankful.

Enjoy the time you spend working with the natural world and observe how it feels along the way. If your crop bears fruit, notice what it's like to eat something that you've nurtured into being. If you can't grow your own, take some time to visit an active farm where you can buy food direct-ly from the source. Community-supported agriculture farms (CSAs) are a great way to find organic produce. In some areas it's possible to find farms that will exchange work for some of the harvest. For further CSA informa-tion, go to the United States Department of Agriculture Website, under Alternative Farming, at *www.nal.usda.gov/afsic/pubs/csa/csa.shtml.*

Review

≫ Nutrition is best thought of as all that we consume for nourishment.

≫ Our food consumption affects our individual self, the natural world, and other people. We can choose to consume in ways that will have a positive effect.

≫ Our culture and individual personality influence our consump-tion. Bring awareness to positive and negative impacts, and make appropriate adjustments.

- One of the best ways to consume with a positive health effect is to eat a whole-food, plant-based diet.
- Fill your plate with a wide variety of colors in order to take in a broad range of nutrients.
- Take appropriate supplements, including a decent multivitamin that contains vitamin B12 and an omega-3 fat supplement.
- Consume at least 80 ounces of clean, purified water daily.
- Stop and calm in order to be fully present while you're eating. Eat mindfully with complete focus on your food instead of multitasking.
- Buy organic for fruits and vegetables that have high pesticide residues like the Dirty Dozen, and buy non-organic for the Clean 15.
- Reduce inflammation in the body by eating whole foods and limiting processed, sugary foods, and animal products.
- Connect with the natural world as the source of your nourishment.

Be aware of your habits and attachments concerning foods and eating; make small adjustments, and be gentle with yourself.

Yoga Bits

- Take a mindful breath before eating or drinking anything.
- Chew your food until it becomes liquid in your mouth.
- Smell your food before eating.
- Eat a meal in silence, either with others or alone. Keep your focus on the food and eating, instead of multitasking.
- Purposefully consume less for one meal.
- Grow your own food, or join a CSA and support organically raised local food production.

STEP 5:
PHYSICAL ACTIVITY

If we could give every individual the right amount of nourishment and exercise, not too little and not too much, we would have found the safest way to health.

—Hippocrates

Our next area of focus is the "energy out" side of the equation and achieving balance with all we take in. If we take in more energy from food than we put out through activity, we'll gain weight because excess energy is stored for later use. This energy balance can also be applied to our mental and spiritual processes.

The value of physical fitness in health maintenance is unquestioned. Physical activity ranges from purely recreational activities to those associated with survival. For most of human existence, physical activity was necessary to gather food, build and maintain shelter, fight wars, and maintain social connections. In the past 150 years, advancing technology has made our day-to-day survival less dependent on body movement. As a result, we've become much more sedentary. Chronic health problems such as diabetes and heart disease, often considered diseases of affluence, have spread widely.

We'll keep our integrative stance and look at all of the factors that contribute to our physical activity. Physical activity is more than just exercise. It includes all actions performed by the body and, despite the term *physical*, also includes the mind and spirit. Let's begin with some definitions.

Exercise is structured, planned, and repeated movement that increases physical capacity and maintains health through flexibility, aerobic capacity, and muscle strength.

In the engineering world, **flexibility** is recognized in designs that adapt to external changes. If a bridge isn't flexible enough to accommodate high winds, it won't last very long. Similarly, earthquake-resistant buildings are designed to adjust to the shifting ground and remain standing. In the human body, flexibility is measured by how the joints move through their full range of motion. When the ligaments and muscles that facilitate joint movement are held too tightly in place, they restrict the range of motion. When this is the case, adapting to external changes becomes difficult. Injury occurs when the range of motion required for a specific action exceeds the body's ability to move. But when muscles are stretched and loose, they're more likely to move the joints safely. Careful stretching of the muscles and ligaments greatly improves flexibility.

Aerobic capacity is measured by how well the heart, lungs, and blood vessels provide oxygen to the body during exertion. Usually, low- to moderate-intensity aerobic movement brings enough oxygen to the muscles to convert stored energy into fuel. If there isn't enough oxygen to meet demand, the activity becomes anaerobic. **Anaerobic** exercise is usually more intense and doesn't depend on oxygen. This lack of oxygen can create lactic acid buildup and microscopic muscle tears. This buildup is what makes you feel sore a couple of days after exercise. Fortunately, the lactic acid dissipates and these small tears are gradually repaired.

In terms of energy use, it's moderate-intensity aerobic exercise that burns the energy stored in muscle tissue, as well as other body reserves such as fat. In fact, it may seem counterintuitive, but the higher the intensity of the exercise, the less fat you burn! Exercising for 30 minutes at two-thirds of your maximum effort level is the best way to burn off stored energy. Table 5–1 shows an estimate of calorie-burning sources for a 20-year-old with a maximum heart rate of 200 beats per minute. **Maximum effort** can be gauged by measuring your heart rate during exercise and referring to Table 5–2. You can measure your heart rate in number of beats per minute by placing your pointer finger just behind your voice box and gently feeling your carotid artery. Count your heart-beats for six seconds and multiply that number by 10. Aerobic capacity can be improved in time by being more physically active.

Intensity (%MHR)	Heart Rate (bpm)	% Carbohydrate	% Fat
65–70	130–140	40	60
70–75	140–150	50	50
75–80	150–160	65	35
80–85	160–170	80	20
85–90	170–180	90	10
90–95	180–190	95	5
100	190–200	100	

Table 5–1: Estimate of Calorie Burning Sources for a 20-year-old With a Max Heart Rate of 200 Beats Per Minute.

Muscle strength relates to a muscle's ability to contract and produce the same effect over time. Some muscles, such as those of the heart and bowels, contract throughout sustained periods of time without any conscious control. These muscles can become stronger and more efficient through aerobic activity. Others, including those of the face, back, neck, chest, abdomen, legs, arms, hands, and feet, contract only with conscious effort. This type of muscle is strengthened when it contracts to move the body against resistance, overcoming a specific force. We know this process as resistance or strength training.

※ ※ ※

It's a good idea to keep all types of physical capacity in mind when making exercise choices. We'll help you discover how much physical activity is appropriate and sustainable for you.

EXERCISE ZONES

Age

BEATS PER MINUTE	20	25	30	35	40	45	50	55	65	70
	200	195	199	185	180	175	170	165	155	150
VO2 Max (Maximum effort)										
	180	176	171	167	162	158	153	149	140	135
Anaerobic (Hardcore training)										
	160	156	152	148	144	140	136	132	124	120
Aerobic (Cardio training/Endurance)										
	140	137	133	130	126	123	119	116	109	105
Weight Control (Fitness/Fat burn)										
	120	117	114	111	108	105	102	99	93	90
Moderate Activity (Maintenance/Warm up)										
	100	98	95	93	90	88	85	83	78	75

Table 5–2: Exercise Zones

First, find a few minutes to focus on the present moment by taking a few conscious breaths or by using a breath-focused exercise. If you become distracted as you read the following pages, bring your attention back to your breath wherever you feel it and then return to the section in front of you. We recommend making notes in your journal or in the margins of this book. Give yourself a few minutes to carefully consider the questions posed for each section. This process will help you determine what type, duration, timing, and frequency of physical activity works best for you.

Physical activity with people and animals

Some activities are best done in groups. For example, the first rule in water safety is never to swim alone. Remember: Exercise should be purposeful and planned; including friends is a great way to help you stick with an exercise plan. Increased daily movement also sets a good example for family and neighbors.

Questions to ponder:

⫸ Are there exercise groups in your area that you'd feel comfortable joining?

⫸ Do you currently exercise with anyone?

⫸ Can you expand that relationship? Are there any barriers?

⫸ Is there a small way you can increase your physical activity and benefit others as well?

Animals can be an important part of life. Are there ways to include pets in your regimen? Are there ways that you can be physically active and benefit animals living in the wild? Collecting harmful trash is one example of helping animals in their natural environment.

Physical activity and the natural world

There is an entire field of study included in public health literature that concerns how to improve the environment and make it more suitable for physical activity. Many factors influence whether individuals are physically active. These include the weather, setting (urban, suburban, or rural), space availability, and access to pedestrian-friendly travel. Take a few minutes to think about your local environment. Consider if there is anything that keeps you from the physical activities that you enjoy and if there are any untapped resources available to you. Make a list of the best activities closest to home. Are there ways you can improve the local environment to provide easier access to these activities?

It's possible for increased physical activity to have a positive influence on the natural world. For example, it happens when we drive less and walk or bike more. What better way to reduce the use of fossil fuels and get healthier in the process! Consider how you can have a positive impact on the natural world and increase your physical activity at the same time.

For millennia, producing food for survival has required hard work. Planting, maintaining, and harvesting fruits and vegetables are excellent ways to combine physical activity with a tangible connection to nature. It also provides fresh, nutritious foods to eat. Many of our group participants mention gardening as a favorite hobby. Gardening can keep us active year-round. Along with fruits and veggies, planting trees, plants, and flowers not only makes the landscape more beautiful, but also produces oxygen for the environment.

Physical activity and culture

The culture in which we're raised heavily influences how we view physical activity. Some cultures view it as a luxury and don't give it a high priority.

Questions to ponder:

» Were you raised to value exercise?

» Does your family focus on competitive sports, ceremonial rituals, or fiestas?

» How does your faith community view physical activity? How is it encouraged, and how is it practiced? Have you faced cultural barriers to physical activity? How can these barriers be addressed?

Physical activity can have a positive cultural influence, especially when it's performed inside common values. What are creative ways to increase physical activity levels inside your culture?

Physical activity and the lens of self

Reflect on your greatest strengths and weaknesses related to your personality type. How do they influence the type of exercise you enjoy? Do you prefer to exercise on your own or in groups? Do you prefer to be spontaneous or do you like to plan ahead? Do you exercise as a part of being social? When you're feeling out of balance, what tends to motivate you the most? Do you tend to over-exercise? Do you enjoy mastering a single activity or dabbling in many?

In addition to the Enneagram, there are other ways to find your fitness personality type. The American Institute for Cancer Research put together a simple quiz to determine whether you tend to be a self-motivator, a team player, or more spontaneous with regard to physical activity. Here it is:

When I think about physical activity, I:
1. Can't wait to put on my walking shoes.
2. Really want to exercise but need a push.
3. Dread the idea of moving a muscle, but am happy once I get moving.

When I am physically active, I enjoy exercising:
1. By myself at my own pace.
2. With a team or group.
3. With one or two buddies.

I exercise because:
1. I want to stay in shape, slim down, or improve my health.
2. I want to see friends and catch up on the latest news.
3. The weather is nice or I just feel like it.

When I take part in a physical activity, I usually:
1. Plan the event ahead of time.
2. Participate when someone else has set up the activity, or attend a class.
3. Pull it together quickly and do something active when the mood strikes.

Others see me as:
1. A leader.
2. A team player.
3. Someone who goes along with a good idea.

I enjoy physical activities that are:
1. Set by my own routine.
2. Set by a professional, teacher, or group.
3. Spontaneous.

Scoring: For every answer of a given number, give yourself:
1 = 1 point
2 = 2 points
3 = 3 points

If you scored...

6–9 points—You are a self-motivator. Self-motivators like to be structured and organized, but may tire of routine. It's a good idea for them to try a variety of activities, mixing things up to stay engaged.

10–14 points—You are a team player. Team players like to be connected with others and do best when they plan workouts in groups or attend exercise classes.

15–18 points—You are spontaneous. Spontaneous individuals prize freedom and dislike rigid schedules or rules.

(The Fitness Personality Quiz is reprinted with permission from the American Institute for Cancer Research)

As we found with the Enneagram, these traits aren't written in stone, but they're helpful tools for the self-understanding needed in planning and maintenance. Take some time to consider this information with regard to what is best for you individually. **Self-motivators** should create a weekly activity calendar, mix up their routine periodically, or try a new Yoga class. From softball to square dancing, **team players** will want to plan activities in which they engage other people. **Spontaneous individuals** prefer to find exercise in a variety of settings, such as walking a new path in the woods or riding a bike through a less familiar part of the neighborhood.

A good friend, Dr. John Pace, likes to emphasize the fact that we often make excuses in order to avoid what we don't like or to embrace things that we really enjoy. He tells his patients to "make an excuse to exercise," rather than making an excuse to avoid it. Find an activity that fits for you, and make it a priority.

Physical activity and the body

The human body is built to be active. All of our muscles, bones, joints, and ligaments evolved to help us survive and thrive in the natural world. Basic survival is much less dependent on physical activity than it was 1,000, 500, 200, or even 100 years ago because of greater access to clean foods, improved public hygiene, and advances in modern medicine (especially vaccinations and antibiotics). For most of us, the effort to put food on the table relies more on interpersonal relationships than hard labor. So how do we best design a practice that gives us the benefit of physical activity when it's no longer associated with how we make a living? How do we continue to thrive when our survival needs are largely addressed through mechanisms outside of our physical control?

The optimal approach to physical activity varies by age and health status. If you're over 40 and haven't been physically active for some time or have health problems, check with your doctor before beginning any exercise program. We'll focus on a foundational and sustainable process here, which includes exercising on all three levels of capacity: aerobic capacity, muscle strength, and flexibility. One way to define your physical activity program is to determine the frequency, intensity, time, and type (FITT) for each category.

A retired nurse gives us a wonderful example of this approach. She carefully chooses activities from each level of capacity that are appropriate for her age, personality, general health, and locale. Brisk walks in a hilly neighborhood as well as lots of gardening provide great aerobic workouts. Twice each week she meets with a small group of friends for resistance training and a good chat. To increase core strength and flexibility, she combines elements from Pilates and Yoga that are just right for her. At 60, she glows with vitality.

Aerobic capacity

Aerobic exercise is recommended five to six days per week. This can be accomplished with the moderate to vigorous intensity achieved by brisk walking. You can measure your heart rate to see if you're working at a level appropriate for your age, or you can gauge your activity by how hard you're breathing. During moderate aerobic activity, you'll break a sweat and should be able to carry on a conversation. During vigorous activity, you won't be able to carry on a conversation without stopping often to catch your breath. Moderate activity includes a fast walk, water aerobics, pushing a lawn mower, or riding a bike. Vigorous activity includes swimming laps, jogging, riding a bike up hills, or playing soccer or basketball.

Even 10 minutes of aerobic activity can have significant health benefits. Try aiming for a total of 30 minutes of activity each day. Sprinkling this amount throughout the day is just as beneficial as doing it all at once—the body doesn't know the difference. You can add a few minutes of aerobics here and there by parking the car farther away from your destination and walking fast to get there; taking brief, fast walks during the day; and walking to and from lunch, or walking before and after eating. Every little bit of exercise really does help.

Thousands of years ago, Hippocrates understood the impact of consistent physical activity on a person's weight. He said that people who are overweight and trying to lose pounds should always sit down to the table to eat when out of breath, and those trying to gain weight should sit to eat when calm and rested.

Flexibility capacity

Working on flexibility several days per week will help prevent injury and improve general performance. It's best to stretch within a mild to moderate intensity level, and you should always be able to carry on a conversation at the same time. Stretch when your muscles and tendons are warm to avoid strain.

Warm up your body with five minutes of brisk walking or jogging in place. Do your aerobic work and then cool down with some stretching. Always stretch both sides of the body and try to target your flexibility practice based on your activities. If you are mainly moving your lower body, as in walking, jogging, playing soccer, or lifting lower-body weights, then focus your stretching from the midsection down. If you are using your upper body, as in swimming, playing basketball, or lifting upper body weights, then focus your stretches on the midsection up. The back and midsection can be thought of as the center or core of our movement. The core muscles are involved in almost every type of activity, and it's wise to stretch them daily.

Stretching a sore, tense muscle is instinctive. Although it may seem counterintuitive, it's actually more effective to stretch the opposite, complementary muscle group to promote relaxation and release in the sore area. This phenomenon is the basis of the therapeutic practice of *strain/ counter-strain*: When one part of the body is in a strained or working position, a complementary area is in a relaxed or counter-strained position. The counter-strained position triggers a relaxation response that can reverse strain and discomfort in the complementary muscle group. By stretching (strain), we try to lengthen the muscle as much as possible, and by relaxing (counter-strain), we shorten it. A flexibility practice not only helps prevent injury, but it can also reduce existing muscle pain and soreness. For example, you can stretch the muscles on the left side of your neck to relieve pain and tightness on the *right side*. Simply drop the right ear gently toward the right shoulder. Take a few breaths in this position, and then slowly bring your head back to center. Observe the results.

The body should always be well supported to prevent overstretching. Avoid bouncing up and down in a stretch, as quick motion can strain the very muscles or ligaments you're trying to lengthen. Remember to warm up! Again, start with five minutes of brisk walking or stepping in place. A former runner suffering from sciatic nerve pain follows this strategy: After months of pain therapy and little relief, she sought the help of a Yoga teacher. Together, they combined a series of gentle and sustained stretches with breath awareness. In only a few sessions, the pain disappeared and freedom of movement returned.

A focus on breathing is essential while stretching. You'll relax more deeply into the stretch by matching gentle effort with the rhythm of the breath. You can usually go deeper into a stretch with the out-breath and rest there in a relaxed way with the in-breath. Use the Stop, Calm, and Rest meditation from Chapter 3 before stretching. If you notice areas of tension or tightness in your body, imagine that you can direct the breath to those areas. You can say to yourself:

I breathe in relaxation and warmth.

I breathe out tightness and tension.

Muscle strength capacity

Strengthening our muscles enables us to perform daily activities that require moving our body weight and lifting, carrying, or pulling objects. Muscle strength is vital for those trying to lose weight and hoping to excel in athletic endeavors. Increasing muscle capacity helps the body to do more, and, consequently, when the body has more muscle mass, it uses more calories. Muscle strengthening can be accomplished with mild- to moderate-intensity exercise and includes daily activities such as lifting groceries, heavy yard work, or climbing stairs. It can also be done with vigorous intensity such that we target a specific muscle group and work it until we can't complete another repetition. An example of vigorous muscle strengthening is doing as many push-ups as possible.

Mild to moderate muscle-strengthening activities are best done almost daily as a part of an active lifestyle. Vigorous activity that targets specific muscle groups and works them to the point of exhaustion can be done twice weekly.

Muscle groups can be divided into three areas: the **core**, which includes the back and abdominal muscles; the **upper body**, which includes the arms and shoulders; and the **lower body**, which includes the legs and pelvic muscles.

Muscle strengthening can be done in several different ways: You can use your own body weight, as in walking stairs or doing push-ups, or use free weights (such as barbells or dumbbells), resistance bands, or tubing. Weight machines are also popular at most gyms.

We'll focus on maintaining balance in the body by beginning with light to moderate muscle strengthening. For this level of activity, we recommend daily strengthening of the core muscles, as well as the upper and lower body. If you would like to do more focused strengthening of these muscle groups, you could do targeted work by increasing weight or repetitions to the point at which your muscles fatigue twice weekly.

Remember to breathe! Bring mindful awareness to whatever you're doing in the present moment. When it comes to muscle strengthening, bring your focus directly to the muscle group that you are working with, and observe how it feels to move your body against resistance. This present-moment focus will help you get to know the strengths and weaknesses of your body, as well as help you prevent injury. First, remember to warm up your muscles with five minutes of moderate aerobic activity, just as you did before doing flexibility exercises.

≫≫ ≫≫ ≫≫

In the following paragraphs we offer a few sample activities for each of the three physical capacities. These specific stretches and exercises may or may not be appropriate for you or your situation; no one knows your body better than you do. This is *your* journey and we are only guides. Whether you're working out with a group of friends or taking an exercise or Yoga class, do only what's beneficial to you. Even an experienced instructor can miss important cues. Listen to your gut feelings. If you're asked to do something that doesn't seem right for you, a polite "no thank you" is very reasonable. Avoid comparing yourself to others and to what you recall of a younger or healthier you.

As you go through the following exercises, you may notice that most mild to moderate types of exercise are optimally done five to six days per week as a part of a healthy lifestyle. This may seem overwhelming, but it can actually be a good way to improve sustainability by trying new tools in new ways and incorporating them mindfully into your daily life. Remember to start small and pay attention to your body. Routinely, be physically active throughout the day, rather than trying to do it all in a single session.

Along with many other benefits, mindfulness can keep us safe by paying attention to how we're breathing to avoid over-exertion. Notice when intensity approaches pain. Give full attention to any activity you're involved in. When in doubt, check with your integrative healthcare provider. Enjoy.

Increasing flexibility

Open door stretch

This is a good introduction to stretching and a great way to relieve a strained lower back. Many of our group participants have had great success with this stretch. It promotes muscle relaxation by the strain/counter-strain principle: The hamstring muscles at the back of the thigh are stretched, while the complementary muscles in the lower back are relaxed.

Find an open doorway where you can lie down completely with your buttocks on the ground. It's best if there is no door in the opening. Imagine a line that runs from the top of your head down to your belly button. Then position yourself so that this line makes a right angle with the doorframe. Place your right heel up on the doorframe and your left leg flat

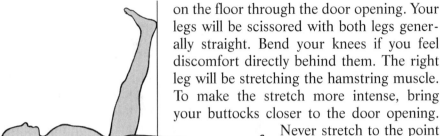

on the floor through the door opening. Your legs will be scissored with both legs generally straight. Bend your knees if you feel discomfort directly behind them. The right leg will be stretching the hamstring muscle. To make the stretch more intense, bring your buttocks closer to the door opening. Never stretch to the point of pain. To increase the stretch, flex your right toes toward the floor. Bring your focus to the hamstring muscle as it stretches, and to the lower back as it relaxes. Breathe into both areas. When you've stretched for 10 breaths or so, repeat on the other side. When you're finished, rest on the floor for a few breaths, and enjoy the relaxation.

Cat stretch

This is a wonderful way to coordinate breathing with movement. Begin on your hands and knees in a neutral tabletop position with your back flat and level with the ground. Place your hands directly under your shoulders and your knees directly under your hips. As you exhale, arch your back up the way a cat would. Allow the top of your head to tip toward the floor as your pelvis curls under. As you inhale, return to a neutral position. Your back may be slightly concave. Follow this wave-like motion for four to five breaths.

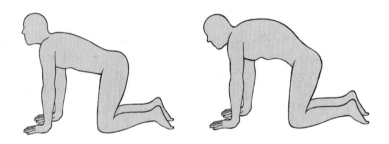

Arm and leg extension stretch

Begin on your hands and knees as you did for the cat stretch, with your back in a neutral position. Focus on the balance between all four points of contact with the floor. Slowly begin reaching your right arm out in front of you. Notice how your balance changes. At the same time, stretch your left leg out behind you. With each exhalation, stretch your arm a little bit farther in front of you and extend the leg farther back. Imagine there is a band gently pulling your arm and leg in opposite directions. As your balance shifts and changes, focus on your breath and contact with the floor. Explore this for several breaths. Rest briefly on all fours before extending the opposite arm and leg. After completing the second side, rest in child's pose (described in the next paragraph) for several breaths.

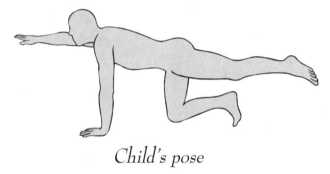

Child's pose

From your position on all fours, slowly let your hips sink back toward your heels. If possible, rest your buttocks on your heels. (If your knees are stiff or uncomfortable, place a rolled towel behind them.) Gently lower your forehead toward the floor, with your arms extended on the floor in front of you. Be here and follow your breath as long as you're comfortable.

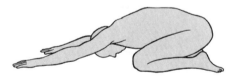

Core muscle strengthening

Arm and leg extension crunches

This builds on the arm and leg extension stretch described in the previous section. With one arm extended forward and the opposite leg extended backward, bring your focus to your balance and your points of contact with the floor. With an exhalation, bend your extended arm and bring your elbow toward your chest. At the same time, bend your extended leg and bring your knee toward your pelvis. With an inhalation, release and extend the arm and leg. Repeat this motion five to 10 times, and then relax in child's pose for a few breaths. Come back to all fours and repeat the exercise with the opposite arm and leg.

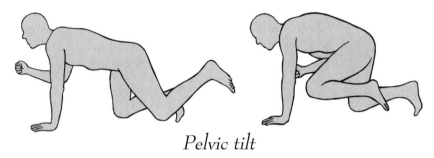

Pelvic tilt

Lie down on your back. Bend your knees and place your feet on the floor directly under your knees, hip width apart. Allow your shoulders to roll back as your arms rest along the side of your body. As your belly sinks back with an exhalation, drop the back of your waist toward the floor even more. Continue breathing as you press down through your heels and curl the pelvis under slightly. Allow your waist to sink into the floor. Release with an inhalation. Allow your pelvis to return to its normal position. Repeat this several times. When you're finished, gently hug your knees toward your chest for a few breaths.

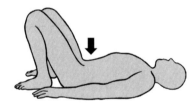

Banana

Begin in the same position you used to begin the pelvic tilt. With an exhalation, straighten your legs and curl your head, neck, and shoulders off the ground, extending your arms toward your feet along the side of your body. From a side view, your body will be shaped like a banana. Hold for two breaths. Relax and curl back down to the ground. Repeat three to four times.

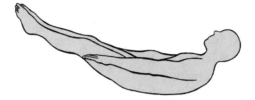

Extended banana

Begin in the same position you used for the banana. With an exhalation, straighten only one leg in front of you and curl your head, neck, and shoulders off the ground, extending your arms toward your feet along the side of your body. Hold for two breaths and return to the ground. Repeat this three to four times and then change legs.

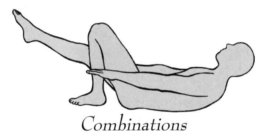

Combinations

Pelvic tilt, banana, and extended banana lend themselves nicely to a continual flow of one movement to another. You can try all of these in sequence for two breaths each. The arm and leg extension stretch can be added for the flexibility portion of your practice.

Upper-body strengthening

Push-ups

Push-ups are a great exercise for strengthening your chest, arm, and shoulder muscles as well as your core. The movement uses your own body weight for resistance as you lower and raise your body to and from the floor. No equipment is needed, although push-up bars may help protect the wrists and also allow for greater range of motion. You can increase or decrease the intensity by varying your leg position. For example, keeping your knees on the floor decreases intensity, whereas lifting one leg in the air or placing both feet on a chair increases intensity.

Start with your body flat on the ground, with your hands along your side, palms on the floor at shoulder level. With an inhalation, tighten your buttocks and abdominal muscles, and lift your body straight toward the ceiling. Your palms and toes support your weight. With an exhalation, slowly bring your body back to the floor. Your chin may touch the floor but your abdomen should not. Repeat for a total of 10 reps. As we mentioned, you can modify the exercise by staying on your knees instead of your toes. You can also modify this by standing and placing your palms on a wall two to three feet in front of you. Then, slowly lower your chest to the wall as you keep your knees and back straight.

Hand positions

To focus on your chest muscles, place your hands wider than shoulder width apart. To target the back and triceps, bring your hands close together with your thumbs and index fingers touching (thumb to thumb, index finger to index finger), making the outline of a triangle in the space between your hands.

Lower-body strengthening

We'll work with the large muscles in the front of the upper legs called the quadriceps as well as the calf muscles in the back of the lower legs. We'll continue our focus on safe exercises that require no equipment.

Sit on the wall

For this exercise find an open space of wall. Place a towel behind your back, and stand with your back flush against the wall. Place your feet about two to three feet in front of you and shoulder-width apart. It's best to do this barefoot or in shoes that don't slide. Slowly slide your buttocks toward the floor. Make sure that your knees do not extend further than your ankles. As you press your back against the wall, lower yourself to as close to a seated position as possible. Don't let your hips sink lower than your knees. Hold this position for three to four breaths. Then slide your back up the wall to a standing position. Rest for a few seconds and repeat two to four times. You should feel this in your thigh muscles.

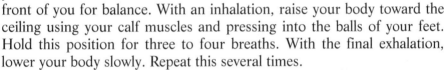

Calf raises against the wall

Stand next to an open space of wall and place your hands on the wall in front of you for balance. With an inhalation, raise your body toward the ceiling using your calf muscles and pressing into the balls of your feet. Hold this position for three to four breaths. With the final exhalation, lower your body slowly. Repeat this several times.

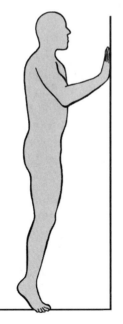

Proper rest

It's vital that you give your body time to rest and recuperate with sleep. As with most things, the right amount varies among individuals. If you wake in the morning and feel rested and ready to go, you're probably getting enough sleep. If you wake in the morning feeling very tired, and remain tired throughout the day, you may need to consider some changes in your sleep-wake cycle.

During deep sleep that is uninterrupted by light, the brain produces the hormone melatonin, which has many positive influences. Melatonin may guard the nervous system against neurodegenerative diseases such as Alzheimer's and may help cancer patients to live longer. When we wake in the morning, the adrenal gland produces cortisol, which gives us a shot of energy to start the day. If you are constantly fatigued or wake up tired, you may want to consult your integrative physician to evaluate your sleep-wake cycle and to screen for associated medical conditions like hypothyroidism and sleep apnea.

A day of rest is important. Some cultures call this a lazy day; others call it the Sabbath. Take one day each week to recharge your batteries. Be careful about taking extended naps; as this could alter your natural sleep-wake cycle. Limit naps to a half hour per day.

Physical activity and the mind

Often we think of the mind-body link as the mind exerting some type of control over the body. But the body can also influence the workings of the mind: Physical activity can improve your mood. Your mood and state of mind influence what you think about being active and how well you adhere to an exercise plan. Many research studies indicate that the link between the mind and the body is so complete that when the body is flexible, active, and strong, so are the workings of the mind.

It's natural to notice breathing changes when we're physically active, and expanding this awareness brings the mind and the body together as one. Enrich your practice with mindful walking, biking, swimming, jogging, or whatever your activities may be.

Also experiment with bringing awareness to the stuff of daily life. Make your household routine more fulfilling by bringing mindful attention to it. Change a "to-do" list into a "to-be" list. Notice how you move and breathe as you complete household chores. Pay attention to how you load the car with groceries or pile garden supplies into the back of the truck. Do you hold your breath as you work? Do you feel sore afterward? Observe how you stand at the sink when washing the dishes or brushing your teeth. Notice how your shoulders, lower back, hips, and knees feel.

We find inspiration in a woman who discovered the link between her chronic neck pain and the time she spent in the car. Gradually, she noticed how she slumped forward in the driver's seat, rounding her shoulders and jutting out her chin. What was her simple, insightful solution? She adjusted the rearview mirror so that using it required better posture!

There is an important connection between the intentions behind our physical activity and the framework in which they're placed. In *The*

Psychology of Winning, Dr. Denis Waitley looked at elite athletes around the world to determine how they became winners. One very important characteristic that rose to the top involved how athletes set goals to achieve optimal performance. He observed that the way athletes approached goals influenced the outcome. One way was to focus on the goal with all of the associated positive, desirable outcomes. The second was to focus on the negative consequences of missing the goal. We either move toward goals driven by enjoyment in the process and final outcome, or we move toward the goal by avoiding what we fear will happen if we don't achieve it.

Dr. Waitley found that people who accomplish their goals more often do so because they focus on the desire to succeed, rather than on the fear of failure. It's important to note that either path will move an individual toward the goal, but the most successful and sustainable path is to move forward with the desire to enjoy life, rather than the fear of suffering as a result of not reaching the goal. When we think about life's journey, this makes sense.

There will always be difficulties and setbacks as well as small victories along the way. We can choose to see difficulties in a positive light: "I know this exercise is difficult, but I'll be better for it." Or we can see things through the fear of failure: "This exercise is difficult, and I hope I don't mess up again." Which way is more sustainable? We'll never reach complete perfection—nor is that our goal—but we all get an A+ just for trying. We have the capacity to enjoy each moment along the way and move forward with positive intention. When we're motivated by the fear of failure, small roadblocks can seem overwhelming. Instead, set realistic goals that can be reasonably accomplished. Little points of success can be fully enjoyed and celebrated.

Try the following visualization exercise:

1. Close your eyes and bring your focus to the breath. Imagine a large movie screen before you. Project onto that screen the image of your physically fit body.

2. Next focus on being inside of your fit body and what it feels like. How will you enjoy all aspects of your life in this state? Experience how wonderful you will feel when you are physically in balance— able to move over distances, flexible, and strong. What does physical health look like? What does it feel like through every filter of experience? Take a few minutes to explore this and the enjoyment of life that it will bring.

3. Open your eyes. Breathe in and out while focusing on how good it feels to breathe. Retain the feeling of physical fitness somewhere inside you. Call on it when you experience obstacles along the way. When you need encouragement, focus on your breath and recall these feelings.

Your enjoyment of life will help you succeed. Celebrate and thank yourself for little steps along the way. When you encounter difficulties, see them as growing points that will bring you closer to your fitness goals and greater enjoyment of life.

Physical activity and the spirit

Yoga, Tai chi, Qigong, and the martial arts include forms of physical activity that are expressions of the spirit. Yoga is probably the most well-known, and American culture has readily absorbed it. You can find all styles and schools of Yoga. However, an explanation of each is well beyond the scope of our book.

The word *Yoga* has its ancient roots in Sanskrit and means "to yoke" or "to unite." Originally, Yoga referred to the union of the individual with the universal, a complete integration of the mind, body, and spirit. It's possible that the physical element of Yoga evolved simply to help yogis or monks sit for prolonged periods in meditation. Many Yoga poses are based on the movements of animals and connect us to the natural world. The movements of the body are united with the breath, and breath is inspired by spirit.

Today, many Yoga practitioners seek its physical benefits yet ignore important subtle aspects, like the breath. Slender, toned bodies appear in pretzel-like poses to advertise everything from cars to yogurt. However, outward appearances may not reflect inner states of being. By over-emphasizing physical attainment, many Yoga students and teachers force themselves into injuries and chronic conditions. When the alignment of body, mind, and spirit is lost, so is the Yoga. The totality of Yoga has an all-embracing quality. When it's approached with awareness and intention, we tend to develop a flexibility of mind and emotions along with looser hamstrings. Yoga is an open path meant to serve each of us, regardless of age or physical condition. The only requisite is a single breath.

In Jewish tradition, the name for God is Yahweh, actually spelled YHWH, making it unpronounceable and pointing to the unknowable mystery of God. It's interesting that saying *Yahweh* actually corresponds to the sound made with the breath. When we breathe in with the mouth open, we hear "Yah," and as we breathe out, "Weh." Try it for a few breaths. This very powerful practice reminds us that the great mystery that created the universe also animates the physical body with every breath.

Practice

Following are two practice samples of exercise sessions with different intensities.

Moderate Intensity

Morning Routine:

These steps are done in order and flow together, beginning with an aerobic warm-up.

Aerobic: five minutes stepping in place

Flexibility: straight leg in open door

Core Muscle Strengthening: pelvic tilts, banana, extended banana; four sets each

Flexibility: cat stretch for 10 breaths. Arm and leg extension stretch, five breaths on each side

Core Muscle Strengthening: arm and leg extension crunches; 10 each side

Upper-Body Strengthening: 10 push-ups with arms shoulder-width apart, toes on floor; 10 push-ups with hands together in front and knees on the floor

Flexibility: child's pose—five breaths

Before Lunch: 10-minute brisk walk

Mid-Afternoon Stress Break at Work: moving meditation stretch

Before Dinner: 10 minutes of yard cleanup, gardening, or a brisk walk

Before Bed: visualize body fitness goal

Milder Intensity

Morning Routine:

Core Strengthening: pelvic tilts in bed, 10 times

Aerobic: walk the dog through the neighborhood for 20 to 30 minutes

Strengthening: five standing push-ups against the wall; continue with "sit on the wall" for one minute

Flexibility: 10 minutes of gentle Yoga stretches, especially of the neck and shoulders

After Lunch:

Aerobic: plant tomatoes and pull weeds in the flowerbed

Late Afternoon:

Flexibility: cat stretch for five breaths

Before Bed:

Relaxation: follow the breath for two to three minutes

Exploration: Meet the body where it is

We rarely appreciate how our body looks and often ignore the miracle of its daily functions. After all, the body isn't some accessory; it's where we live. It carries us through life and holds our stories in every cell. Mindful awareness can help us stretch beyond our rigid notions of how the body should or shouldn't be. Use the following practice to meet your body *how* and *where* it is, with greater self-acceptance.

1. Find a quiet place. It might be at home or at the office, in your parked car or on a garden bench.

2. Sit down straight and bring your awareness to the breath as it moves through the body.

3. Let go of anything you'd like to let go of to be more fully present. Here and now.

4. Follow the gentle rhythm of your breath. Give your attention to the physical sensations of breath. Simply inhale and exhale.

5. Invite your awareness to expand and wander through your body. Allow your focus to flow to any physical sensations that pull your attention away from the breath.

6. Notice any tightness, itching, tingling, soreness, or pain. Notice the sensations without judgment. Release your opinions about them.

7. Observe the sensations as if they no longer belong to you. Let go of any assumptions or fears about how your body feels. Just feel.

8. Explore the sensations with curiosity. Notice where they start and stop. Meet them with acceptance and understanding.

9. Imagine touching the sensations with tenderness. Hold them as you'd hold the hand of a small child.

10. When you feel ready, release the sensations and return to the flow of your breath. Be with the breath.

11. Begin to deepen your breathing, and slowly come back to the world around you.

12. Gently open your eyes.

Review

We can create a consistently renewing physical activity practice for ourselves with continuous reflection on all parts of this process. This will be filled with the constant adjustments that come through mindful awareness of how we incorporate body movements into our daily lives. We can succeed in our fitness goals and at the same time live fully in the present moment non-judgmentally. It must be a both/and type of process in order to be sustainable: We *both* live in the present moment *and* move toward a goal in the future, motivated by the desire to succeed.

Here's a short checklist to guide you on your way:

» Reflect on your personality and fitness type.

» Set reasonable goals with clear intention.

» Find activities you enjoy.

» Start with something simple.

» Gradually increase your effort.

» Do things at your own speed.

» Get outside.

- ⫸ Build new habits step-by-step.
- ⫸ Be gentle and persistent.
- ⫸ Schedule activities with friends.
- ⫸ Accumulate activities through the day.
- ⫸ Be patient and celebrate small improvements.
- ⫸ Keep yourself safe with mindful awareness.
- ⫸ Let Spirit move you.

Yoga Bits

- ⫸ Explore neck stretches or shoulder rolls for three conscious breaths while sitting in the office.
- ⫸ Explore shifting your weight from one foot to the other while standing in line.
- ⫸ Walk mindfully—counting your steps for each in-breath and out-breath.
- ⫸ Alternately tense and relax specific muscle groups throughout the day.
- ⫸ Plan to scan the body at specific times during the day, looking for any areas of tension. When you find an area of concern, stretch the opposite muscle to provide relaxation, or simply imagine breathing into that area.
- ⫸ Use a physical movement to relax the body and calm the mind. Count eight in-and-out-breaths by using the hands. Touch the finger to the thumb for each of the four fingers on each hand. Simply follow the breath without changing it.

STEP 6:
STRESS MANAGEMENT

Between stimulus and response there is a space. In that space is our power to choose our response. In our response lies our growth and our freedom.

—Viktor Frankl

Stress is a natural part of life. In physics, stress is a force that acts on a specific object and causes deformation or strain. In its application to health and wellness, stress is seen as a force that causes mental, emotional, physical, or spiritual strain. Endocrinologist Hans Selye is considered by many to be the scientific father of the modern idea that stress has a significant effect on living organisms. Dr. Selye described the different types of stress as well as the range of reactions to it. He was the first to determine that stress affects us whether it's considered good or bad, positive or negative.

He defined **eustress** (pronounced "you-stress") as healthy stress that gives one a feeling of fulfillment and enjoyment or enhances physical and mental functions in some way. The Greek root *eu* means "well" or "good"; thus, *eu-stress* is good stress. Examples of eustress include strength training, challenging work, getting married, riding a roller coaster, and experiencing the holidays. Eustress includes positive, healthy gains such as increasing enjoyment and capacity for life, and making meaningful connections with yourself and others.

Distress, on the other hand, is persistent stress that goes beyond our ability to respond. This word originated from the Latin *districtus*, meaning "divided in mind." Distress can't be resolved through coping or adapting. This chronic, unresolved stress can lead to anxiety, withdrawal, and many other physical and emotional problems. Examples include repeated and irreconcilable challenges at work, at home, or in other relationships. It's important to note that both types of stress affect the mind, body, and spirit, and they can add up in time depending on how we respond.

Scientists Thomas Holmes and Richard Rahe took these ideas further and developed the Social Readjustment Rating Scale, now called the Holmes and Rahe Stress Scale. Their scale lists stressful life events and gives them a numerical score. Holmes and Rahe showed that higher scores predict a greater chance that stress will lead to disease. It's important to realize that the scale includes examples of positive eustress as well as negative distress. It shows that stress levels significantly increase with multiple events happening at the same time and demonstrates that mind, body, and spirit do not differentiate between positive and negative stress.

Here is the scale for your review.[1] Use it as a way to focus your awareness on these types of events and the areas of your life they are affecting. To measure stress using this scale, add the number of "Life Change Units" that apply to events within the past year of your life. The final score gives a rough estimate of how stress influences the risk of developing an illness. If your score is very high, it's important to realize that it doesn't sentence you to illness. Basically, this scale points out that any change is stressful and can throw us out of balance, especially if we are not aware.

Picture yourself sitting on your three-legged stool of health, with different parts of the stool affected by the stresses listed in the following table. Change will throw us out of balance in some way. This is why it's so important to meet change when we are calm and at rest. It's vital to stop and cultivate awareness as much as possible so we are aware of how our life is being influenced. Small adjustments can help us sustain balance through change. Change is inevitable, and balance is possible through awareness. Small, well-matched tools used intentionally can promote balance and prevent illness and disease.

Life Event	Life Change Units
Death of a spouse	100
Divorce	73
Marital separation	65
Imprisonment	63
Death of a close family member	63
Personal injury or illness	53
Marriage	50
Dismissal from work	47
Marital reconciliation	45
Retirement	45
Change in health of family member	44
Pregnancy	40
Sexual difficulties	39
Gain a new family member	39
Business readjustment	39
Change in financial state	38
Death of a close friend	37
Change to different line of work	36
Change in frequency of arguments	35
Major mortgage	32
Foreclosure of mortgage or loan	30
Change in responsibilities at work	29
Child leaving home	29
Trouble with in-laws	29
Outstanding personal achievement	28
Spouse starts or stops work	26
Begin or end school	26

Change in living conditions	25
Revision of personal habits	24
Trouble with boss	23
Change in working hours or conditions	20
Change in residence	20
Change in schools	20
Change in recreation	19
Change in church activities	19
Change in social activities	18
Minor mortgage or loan	17
Change in sleeping habits	16
Change in number of family reunions	15
Change in eating habits	15
Vacation	13
Christmas	12
Minor violation of law	11

Score of 300+: At risk of illness

Score of 150–299+: Risk of illness is moderate (reduced by 30 percent from the above risk)

Score of 150 or less: Slight risk of illness

Further scientific studies began to define exactly how stress causes illness. A new discipline called psychoneuroimmunology emerged as data poured in that showed the mind and the body interact in measurable ways. For example, the immune system functions poorly after periods of severe stress. As the name of the field implies, the mind, nervous system, and immune system are interrelated. This field also produced data revealing that the mind and the body are actually one unit, and that the mind is not only located in the brain: Some receptors in the brain that allow the nerves to perform certain actions are also present in immune system cells and even in the lining of the gut. This discovery gives scientific meaning to our intuitive "gut feeling." The gut actually feels and thinks in ways similar to the brain.

Most of us would agree that chronic, unrelenting stress can lead to distress, or bad stress. This can lead to continued unaddressed imbalances, which can then lead to illness and dis-ease. We can easily identify the major events listed in the Holmes and Rahe scale, but what about the small events that stress us out during the day? The red traffic light that seems ridiculously long, small affronts from others, distressing thoughts and feelings—these are everyday occurrences that also add up in time. In short, we know that:

>> Stress is a natural and often beneficial part of life.

>> Making positive health changes is stressful at first.

>> Our reactions to stressful events play an important role in how they affect us.

Questions to ponder:

>> How much stress is too much for you?

>> How can you adapt to change and stressful events, using eu-stress to help you grow, while reducing the accumulation of chronic distress that leads to illness?

>> How do you keep a healthy balance?

PQRRS

Let's take another approach to stress management: **PQRRS— Practice, Question, Reframe, Respond, and Surrender**.

Practice is defined by your intention to cultivate awareness. Being aware of what's happening in your life creates the opportunity to choose your response instead of reacting from previous conditioning. By learning how to stop, calm, and rest, we can bring our focus to whatever is going on in the present moment. It's best to look at areas of our life that can provoke fear (those areas that we would rather dismiss or judge as too difficult to sit with) when we are in a state of rest. When a storm comes up, we first move indoors, making sure that we are safe and warm, and then we can enjoy watching it from a restful place.

Questioning includes bringing your focused awareness to life events, thoughts, and concerns with gentle curiosity and observing your automatic reactions. This is like a newborn baby just brought into the home: When the baby cries, the parent goes to the baby and tries to figure out what he or she needs. The parent doesn't rush in and immediately change the diaper. The parent will usually hold the baby, rock him or her gently, and try to understand what it needs. Is the baby hungry, wet, sick, or scared? Then the parent uses the right technique for the best response.

When we are aware of what's happening in our life—what pushes our buttons and what happens when those buttons are pushed—we can begin to hold our automatic reactions as the focus of our awareness, much like holding a crying baby. We can hold the baby of our anger, for instance, and ask where it came from. What caused the anger to show up? What watered the seeds of our anger in the past, and how does it relate to the present situation? Through questioning, we can gain some understanding, and through understanding, we can gain insight.

This insight helps us **Reframe** how we look at things. It is easier to water the seeds of compassion when we take a more complete perspective. Reframing is the power behind the WWJD bracelets asking "What Would Jesus Do?" Taking the perspective of your highest and best self, or of a trusted mentor, is a good way to see a situation in a new light. Often, this is enough to change the chronic accumulation of distress into life-enhancing and temporary eustress.

With reframing, we can choose to **Respond** in ways that no longer water unpleasant and distressing seeds. Our thoughts and actions begin to water life-affirming seeds in ourselves and others. We respond in ways that are grounded in understanding, rather than reacting in ways that avoid our fears. A group member's drawing of a closed door in a dark room represented what held her back. She was afraid to open the door and afraid to stay stuck in the dark. The light of awareness allowed her to see turning the door handle as an opportunity to confront what waits on the other side. She moved forward with understanding, rather than remaining immobilized with fear.

Once we respond, the next step is to **Surrender** our control over whatever happens next. We don't know what's on the other side of the door, but we choose to move forward and open it anyway. The other side will certainly contain something, but we can't know what it will be beforehand. Addressing our fears, meeting life with understanding, and watering positive seeds doesn't necessarily mean that doing so will bear fruit that we'll deem immediately positive. It also doesn't mean that others will always respond positively to our actions. We don't respond in order to get something specific in return. We choose the best response based on our understanding and compassion for ourselves and all that's involved in the process.

Surrendering sets us free from "us versus them" thinking and allows us to remain open to whatever happens in this moment and the next. Surrendering helps us give up our attachment to some desired outcome. Often our attachment to the positive or aversion to the negative can keep us stuck in the dark, afraid to move forward and meet new challenges.

Put PQRRS to the test during some of your quiet time. As you become stronger in your awareness practice, it will be easier to focus and question deeply without thoughts and worries distracting you. You're training your mind to maintain focus and slow the habit energy that bounces from one thought, feeling, or situation to another. This mental habit isn't something to eliminate, but something to observe as a potential teacher. Why do particular thoughts occur over and over again? Where do they come from? One helpful practice is to name these recurring thoughts. For example: "Oh, there's my old friend insecurity [anger, jealousy, or other] coming to visit again. Why are you here? Where did you come from, and what's giving you energy in my life?" Often this process can provide insight into whatever we're facing. If a particular situation brings up these "old friends," consider the source. If and when you lose focus on a particular question, consciously let go of whatever grabs your attention. Recognize it as just another thought, and bring your awareness back to the breath. Then, return to the question and wait for further understanding and insight.

Stressful events have different timing. Stressors can be immediate, short-term, or long-term. Using the PQRRS practice will help you cope with many types of stressors. You'll also notice a pattern in how you react to stress. Once you recognize your patterns and general tendencies, you can find a way to balance things out. For example, if you tend to slow down and isolate with stress, some group-oriented physical activity may be beneficial. If you tend to get hyped up and overly active, a meditation or Yoga practice may be useful.

The reframing aspect of the three-legged stool of health

An important characteristic of the stress-management leg of our three-legged stool of health is the potential to reframe almost any situation. Nearly every stressful event in life can have a distinct positive and negative impact. In stress management, the individual's perception and experience of the stress makes all of the difference. Notice how we're not using the term *stress reduction*, because the only way to reduce the stress of life is to withdraw from it. The ultimate stress reduction is lack of life. We use the word *management* instead to emphasize our ability to respond with awareness and avoid chronic, unrelenting distress while embracing life-enhancing eustress. What's distress for one individual may be eustress for another. For example, some people like bungee jumping off bridges, whereas others would consider it very distressing with no positive rewards.

Stress management is different from the other two legs of the stool in this regard. With nutrition, for example, nothing is going to make the daily consumption of large amounts of alcohol good for you just because you look at it differently. In physical activity, a total lack of movement is not optimal just because you frame it in a certain way. In stress reduction, the way that an individual sees and experiences a certain event can help determine whether it's eustress or distress. Our point of view is a powerful tool.

Remaining open to the possibility of reframing, let's proceed with our integrative process, making sure to include all aspects of our being and experience. We'll hold questions in mind about stress and how it affects us. And we'll use a stable reference to help examine how we choose to see stress in various parts of our life.

The present moment—enjoying stability

Use the meditation presented on pages 88 and 89. It can establish that firm frame of reference in the present moment and also helps emphasize that our stable enjoyment of life can have a major impact on whether we see life events as eustress or distress. It's a good thing to be stable and calm enough that we can find joy in simply breathing in and out. This can help us enjoy the fact that we are alive, even in the face of challenges. Let's proceed and look at how stress affects all levels of our being and experience.

Stress management and all participants

Humans are social beings. Sharing time with friends and family can be a significant stress management tool, and can also be a source of eustress or distress, depending on the situation. Stress tends to be relational. Some individuals we come into contact with will cause distress and some will be sources of eustress. Consider which individuals in your life help you cope with stress and which ones cause it.

Questions to ponder:

- » How does your family manage stress in general?
- » How do you think your family members learned how to manage stress?
- » How do your work colleagues manage stress? How do they create it?
- » Are there possibilities for increased understanding and forgiveness with family and friends? What barriers would restrict you from this?

Sometimes personal relationships require us to look with mercy and awareness at painful and deeply buried feelings. It can be helpful for yourself and the other person to write a letter of forgiveness. A sample letter is found in the Resources section on page 226. Even unsent, the letter can be very healing. To write this letter, set aside some quiet time and space, and start with the Stop, Calm, and Rest meditation. Think of whatever action, thought, or event caused you pain. Use the PQRRS method. Bring the action, thought, or event into your focused awareness. Ask yourself how it made you feel, and what may have motivated the other person in this situation. Is there a way for you to reframe the event in a way that makes it life-enhancing? Next, write down whatever your practice reveals. Do this without judgment. Close by surrendering your attachment to whether or not this process will have any effect. Keep the letter to come back to, repeating the same exercise several times.

Ultimately, the goal for managing stress is finding the ability to share your life with others in ways that promote joy and decrease suffering. The letter-writing exercise using the PQRRS framework may or may not lead to sending an actual letter. When we address long-held, stressful life events, their hold over us is lost, and we are free to move forward.

Stress management and the natural world

The natural world provides the backdrop to life. If our life is truly like a play, then the natural world offers us all of the scenery, the stage, and the many supporting characters. Whereas we can take refuge in nature to relax and renew, our environment can also cause significant distress. Environmental stresses come to us in various forms of pollution involving light, sound, air, water, space, and time.

Light pollution exists when harsh, artificial lights are constantly on in the buildings where we work and in the natural world outside. Darkness has an important physiologic function, as it stimulates the brain to produce melatonin during the prolonged darkness of sleep. If we are exposed to any kind of light during sleep, melatonin levels drop, and this can have adverse health effects. Night-shift workers often have problems with light exposure and are also found to have a greater chance of developing breast cancer. Light pollution may be one reason for this. Excess use of artificial light can also produce increased anxiety and stress. There is a reason why movies will show scenes in which someone is being questioned with a bright light shining in his or her eyes. Take some time to reflect on how light pollution is present in your daily experience and how you can address it. If possible, enjoy the night sky away from constant city lights. Gently gaze at the stars twinkling in distant darkness.

Sound pollution includes excessive and unpleasant noise that disturbs our actions and thoughts. Excess noise from airplanes, trains, and cars is commonplace. This type of pollution can affect the health of humans and wildlife in a variety of ways, including manifesting as hearing loss, poor sleep, and increased anxiety levels. Much work is being done to lessen human-made noise pollution through better planning and sound-dampening methods, such as the large walls on the sides of major highways that border residential neighborhoods. Are there any distressing types of noise pollution in your daily life? How do you manage these disruptions? Drop a sound-focus meditation into your day. Passively listen to the sounds in your environment without judgment or trying to figure out where they're coming from. Just listen. Try this for a few minutes.

Air and water are two of our most important natural resources and certainly affect our health. When pollution compromises these vital resources, there may be added physical and mental stress. How are **air and water pollution** levels in your area monitored? What can you do to help clean and maintain a natural environment? Clean, fresh air and water can also provide relaxation and enjoyment. Take some time to savor the aroma of the woods and the crisp taste of clean water.

Time crunches and **inadequate space** also contribute to the stress in our lives. Long daily commutes to work, disorganized work areas, excessive work hours, and too many responsibilities quickly and adversely affect the quality of life.

Questions to ponder:

- ⋙ How do you get to and from home and work?
- ⋙ Look at the environments in which you live and work. Are they promoting stress? What can you do to soften their impact?
- ⋙ Is it time for a spring cleaning to lessen clutter?
- ⋙ Are there ways for you to share responsibilities at work or home to create more time?
- ⋙ Look at an entire page from your daily calendar. Do your actions match your priorities in life?

Find small gaps for a few minutes of rejuvenation time, perhaps noticing the breath, or doing some mindful stretching.

Of course, our environment can also have a very positive impact on our health. We are meant to thrive in a natural world of parks and forests, open spaces filled with healthy natural light, calming sounds, and clean streams, lakes, and air. Human schedules don't govern nature. Sitting silently in nature, walking through a park, smelling a flower, and enjoying the companionship of pets are all enjoyable activities with calming health benefits. Nature can teach us about life in general, if we take the time to look. By observing the interconnection of the trees, shrubs, grasses, insects, and animals, we sometimes see the areas of balance and imbalance in our own lives more clearly.

Heather shares a lesson learned in her garden:

Our daily walk was finished. My dog and I returned from taking our usual path in our usual pattern. We approached the front door, and as I turned my key in the lock, my dog became startled and backed away slightly. She drew my gaze down to the doormat and pointed her nose at a rather large tarantula wedged between the mat and the door.

Everything my son taught me about tarantulas came flooding into my head: They're pretty gentle and rarely bite. If they do bite, it feels something like a bee sting. They can live a very long time; they're more fragile than they look; some of them are pink.

And there it was at my front door. What if it crawled into the house when I opened the door? What if someone stepped on it? What if it sunk its fangs into my dog's nose? The lizards, toads, and frogs living in our garden are familiar and expected. But this creature was...well, a little scary. Even so, it had to be rescued. And wouldn't a 10-year-old boy love to see it?

With gloved hands I carefully scooped up the tarantula. Immediately, it drew eight hairy legs close to its body and made itself smaller in the palm of my hand. I found my breath, and began to study her. As my hand relaxed, so did the tarantula. I gently placed her in a box and formed a makeshift habitat around her. She'd be comfortably confined until David got home from school. I could hardly wait.

David smiled as soon as he saw her and said she was awesome. He nodded with approval as I told my story. We wondered how long she'd been living in the garden and if there were others. Wise beyond his years, he said, "It's time to let her go." He chose a spot near some rocks and a big agave, and set the box down on the ground. We very carefully tipped it on its side to give our tarantula full view of the garden, expecting her to scurry out. But she didn't. She held on to the side of the box.

I checked on the tarantula many times that afternoon. Free to go, she sat just inches from her natural habitat. With the whole garden in front of her, why did she stay in the box? Finally, David said, "Mom, you need to stop now. She has to find her own way out. It's up to her." Of course, he was right. And the next morning, the tarantula was gone.

With that new day, I recognized the similarities between the tarantula and myself. Like her, I can peer out from a protected corner, stubbornly attached to the way things are. And I recalled the times I've clung to something well beyond my own best interests. Like the tarantula, I've taken shelter in awkward places just steps from a greater freedom.

I'm grateful for my afternoon with the tarantula. Along with bittersweet memories, her presence brought back powerful lessons. I'm reminded that there are times when holding on to something makes us more vulnerable than letting it go. The tension of resisting change can be more stressful than embracing it. And there really is a garden all around us, when we step forward for a fuller view.

Stress management and culture

The prevailing attitudes in our culture about balancing work and life can have a significant impact on us. In American culture, individuals are often identified by the work they do, and their value to society is measured by the amount of money they make. Some professional fields require nearly complete self-neglect outside of work in order to excel. Medicine, many corporate leadership positions, and the legal world are among them. This type of emphasis is not usually found in Eastern cultures, where family relations are more highly valued. There are also differences in the way that specific cultures perceive stress. What is considered eustress in one culture may be distressing in another. Cultural backgrounds often dictate what kind of coping strategies are used and appropriate ways for individuals to seek out help. For example, it's common for individuals in Eastern countries to live with their extended family under one roof. This arrangement can serve as a great coping resource. In Western countries, where this is rare, elderly family members are more often seen as potential burdens than resources. Dr. Matt often shares during group sessions that his oldest son's first sentence was "Need help." The childlike innocence and humility that requests help when needed is often lost as we age.

Questions to ponder:

» How do your family, work, and culture influence how you manage stressful life events?

» How does your culture teach you to seek help when you have distress?

» Are there ways to manage stress that you're not taking advantage of?

Stress management and the lens of self

The Enneagram teaches us that different personality types have specific basic fears and desires. Our health and balance in life influence how we express our personality. Certainly, our personality type influences how we manage stress. Take a few minutes here to review your dominant personality type's basic fear and desire.

Automatic reactions to situations can shield us from our basic fears and deny us the opportunity to meet them with awareness. Knee-jerk actions also keep us from moving closer to our basic desires and toward expressing our virtues. When we respond to life with awareness and express our greatest strengths, our individual benefit expands to those around us.

As a further exploration, think about a recent major stressor in life. You can choose one that is listed on the Holmes and Rahe scale if nothing immediately comes to mind.

Questions to ponder:

» How did this situation affect you?

» How did you address the situation?

» If you experienced this with another individual, can you step back and see how he or she addressed the situation?

» What was the most difficult part of the process for you?

» How did your actions line up with your basic fear and desire?

» Are there lessons here that can increase self-understanding and prepare you to cope with future stressors?

By understanding our "personal standard operating procedures" we can cultivate awareness of our reactions to stress. When we find ourselves reacting, it can be a cue to stop and question, reframe, respond, and surrender.

Stress reduction and the body

Has anyone ever told you that you need to get out of your head as a way to relieve stress? The body can be a significant source of eustress and distress. Eustress can include sexual activity, hobbies, exercise, and recreational activities such as skiing or skating. These very same activities could lead to distress for some individuals if taken to their extremes, such as promiscuity, extreme sports, bungee jumping, and so on. Often when we are under stress, we tend to move toward extremes, either under- or overemphasizing the physical body.

Physical activity has a definite impact on mental and emotional states, and physical regimens are among recommended therapies for reducing stress, anxiety, worry, and depression. Being active increases the "feel-good" chemicals in your brain called endorphins—which are responsible for the runners' high, for instance. Exercise can improve sleep, increase self-confidence, and, when it's approached with mindful awareness, become a moving meditation. Exercise can distract you from dominant thoughts and worries, and can make it easier to see things from a different perspective.

There are also several body-focused techniques that can help to reduce distress and improve well-being. **Progressive muscle relaxation** is an outstanding method that you can use on your own. It can be especially helpful prior to sleep. Basically, you begin at the top of your head and progress through your body down to the tips of your toes, alternately tensing and relaxing each muscle group.

Here's a mini exercise to practice muscle relaxation:

Start with a conscious breath, in and out. Then purposefully tense up all of the muscles in your body below the waist. Hold this tension for two breaths, and then actively release the tension and relax the muscles, breathing into them for five breaths. Then, tighten up your abdominal and chest muscles for two breaths. Relax and release this tension for five breaths. Next, actively tense the muscles of your arms for two breaths. Relax and release for five breaths. Finally, clench down the muscles of your jaw for two breaths. Relax and release for five breaths. During the process notice how different the muscle groups feel after tensing and relaxing. You may want to finish the exercise with watching your breath for a few minutes to enjoy the sensations of body-wide relaxation.

Massage is a practice that can offer stress relief and improve anxiety, and often offers a caring connection with the person giving the massage. Massage is best given by a licensed therapist, familiar with a variety of techniques. Therapists can use a light, gentle touch or deep-pressure techniques. For stress reduction, gentle forms of massage are probably best, such as a Swedish massage. If you have certain areas of muscle tightness or soreness, deep tissue, sports massage, or focusing on painful trigger points may be helpful.

Trusted family members or friends can also learn to give a gentle massage. In his DVD, *Touch, Caring and Cancer*, William Collinge offers a simple method for giving massages to loved ones living with cancer. This program includes step-by-step instructions for caregivers. The basic steps include a centering exercise, a statement of positive intention for healing, and light massage techniques. It's striking how often caregivers comment that giving a massage made them feel good because it allowed them to offer care and compassion in a concrete way.

Yoga, **Tai chi**, and **Qigong** are mindful methods of moving the body that can have multiple stress-reduction benefits. There are many styles and forms of these practices, and the way they're presented is greatly influenced by the training and experience of the instructor. It's important to shop around for a good match that fits your needs.

Food and stress

The food you're putting into your body can also affect your stress levels. Are you eating or drinking food with significant amounts of sugar and caffeine? When you are stressed, do you drink alcohol to calm down? These substances may increase anxiety and stress, and decrease sleep quality. Rather than using these substances to help us slow down or speed up, it's better to carefully choose tools that affect us in a natural way.

A good alternative to using food to address stress is breath-focused relaxation. Dr. Andrew Weil recommends relaxed breathing to help calm down quickly. You breathe in for a count of four, hold for a count of seven, and then exhale for a count of eight. Repeat for a total of four cycles. With any technique, it's important to stay in your comfort zone. If you become dizzy or lightheaded, or feel any discomfort, return to your normal breathing pattern. A further exercise for breath-focused relaxation can be found at the end of this chapter.

Stress management and the mind

When most people think of the word *stress*, it usually defines an experience centered in the mind. Where is the mind? Is the mind the same thing as the brain? The mind is the part of us that interprets experience and manages responses to internal and external stimuli. As we learned from the science of psychoneuroimmunology, the nervous system is everywhere in the body, not just in the brain. We are a whole interactive system. From an integrative perspective, higher levels of wholeness always include lower levels. For example, a liver is a complete, whole organ, but it cannot exist without the less comprehensive liver cells, or without the microscopic parts of those cells. Higher levels of organization always transcend and include the lower levels. It is a *both/and*, not an *either/or* proposition. This is one way to distinguish a healthy, balanced, higher level of function from one that is unsustainable and unbalanced.

The mind is a whole system that includes the nervous system, but it's not limited to it. The mind includes conscious and unconscious aspects. The conscious mind includes how we choose to respond to events as they unfold. The unconscious mind governs reactions to events as they are colored by past conditioning, previous experience, automatic judgments, and expectations. Further, the unconscious mind contains all of the seeds of experience that have existed for millennia as a part of being human. Psychologist Carl Jung called this part of the mind the collective unconscious.

Let's return to our garden metaphor. The soil of the mind contains the seeds of every possible human emotion, role, action, and thought that has ever been (the collective). When we are born, we each have some seeds that are already stronger than others, which give us a dominant personality type. As we grow, certain seeds are watered more than others. Patterns develop that may cause our reactions to life to become automatic and unconscious. With practical application of awareness, we can weed out our automatic reactions, and bring our conscious mind to the forefront, to use the whole wealth of our available knowledge and experience. As we find the freedom to choose our responses, we are transformed from unconscious doers into conscious beings. We do not get rid of the unconscious mind; it's transcended and included in a bigger whole that includes both the unconscious and the conscious mind. The larger whole includes reactions and responses, as appropriate.

Working with the mind

There are many useful techniques that can help us turn distress into eustress and cope with stresses beyond our control. Hobbies are things that we naturally enjoy doing and are one way of reframing our perspective. When we're absorbed in them, time and performance pressures vanish and we drop into the flow of just being. When we're in the flow of being, the color of our flower of expression influences all of the other flowers in the vase of our life. Our being influences and pervades all of our doing.

The techniques found in **meditation**, **visualization**, and **imagery** offer a wide variety of options for relaxation. **Meditation** finds its roots as a spiritual tool in many spiritual, religious, and cultural traditions. Only recently has it been considered useful for stress management. Meditation usually involves focusing on a specific thing, such as your breath. For stress management, this helps us become aware of what is going on, and, as we train our mind and sharpen our ability to focus, we develop a greater ability to concentrate. With improved focus comes the ability to hold specific questions in mind, leading to deeper understanding and insight.

We then use that insight to limit our suffering and increase life enjoyment for ourselves and others. Mindfulness meditation is the form that we use most in our work, but there are other forms to be explored.

Visualization and imagery involve seeing images with the mind's eye that may facilitate an internal experience. Creative visualization is used often in sports. For example, an athlete would mentally rehearse the perfect race and imagine the experience on every possible level. Some research shows that visualization may improve performance by mentally training muscle memory. Guided imagery sessions usually involve a teacher leading a group or an individual through a situation with visual prompts in order to cultivate insight. Guided imagery usually focuses on relaxing images, such as a favorite place in nature, and provides a setting of safety and rest in which to explore parts of our life that have been previously dismissed. Guided imagery can also be used to promote relaxation during otherwise-stressful situations, such as imagining you are lying on the beach during an MRI scan.

Please try the following guided imagery exercise:

- Find a quiet, comfortable space to lie down. Take a minute or two to settle back and relax. Gently close your eyes.

- Imagine lying directly against the sand on a perfectly beautiful beach. Invite yourself to rest in this place, safe and protected. Give the weight of your body to the ground as completely as you can. Your body becomes so relaxed and heavy that it makes a very deep impression in the sand beneath you. Feel the sensations of release. Allow yourself to be cradled by the Earth. Be here as the breeze moves softly against your skin and the sun gently warms you. Hear the water gently lapping the shore. Enjoy being here, moment by moment. Imagine.

- Surrender any remaining tension and begin to follow the wave-like movement of your breath deep inside. Each breath flows into the next. Each wave of breath dissolves into a sea of awareness. Witness this ebb and flow. Take refuge here, safe and protected. Rest every part of your body, mind, and spirit. Rest.

- As you feel ready, gradually open your eyes. Move and stretch your body as it needs to. Come back into the room.

- Return to your favorite place, your sanctuary, as often as you need, even for a few breaths. It's as close as your very next thought.

This exercise can be used in stressful situations in order to remain calm, such as when undergoing a medical procedure. It can also be helpful if you have trouble sleeping. If you'd like to explore fears or worries, you can add images to bring these fears and worries into the scene and imagine releasing them into the environment. You can let your troubles float away into the sea, or rise out of your hands like small, helium-filled balloons. For individuals who easily visualize, this can be a very powerful technique. Use your creativity. You may want to record your own imagery session and play it back for yourself. Check our Website, *www.sustainablewellnessonline.com*, for more imagery exercises.

Stress management and the spirit

Multiple links have been found between an active spiritual practice and a reduction of worry and anxiety. Practicing with a community of similar individuals can also provide needed social support during periods of distress. A practice centered on the spirit generally gives meaning to life. When we have a *why* to live, we can tolerate almost any specific *how*. The locus of control in life is often given to a higher power. Reframing events is also made possible through the belief in a higher plan. Trust in a higher power loosens our attachment to outcome and allows for surrender: "Let go and let God."

Living with uncertainty is a capacity of the human spirit. The spiritual practice of prayer can strengthen this capacity. There are two general kinds of prayer: asking prayer and contemplative prayer. Both types can help us to navigate life's uncertainties. **Asking prayer** uses words and phrases such as "Help me," "Guide me," "Allow me," "Give me the strength to," and so on. **Contemplative prayer** opens a channel, or connection, bringing the spirit inside of us in touch with the Spirit that everything shares. Asking prayer puts us in a position in which we are speaking. Contemplative prayer brings us to a place where we listen. Both types of prayer have their role.

The following practice combines asking prayer with contemplation:

» Think about the major stresses in your life right now.

» Using asking language, take a few minutes to write a prayer to support you in managing this stress.

» Then take some time to stop, calm, and rest in whatever way you prefer.

⫸ Offer your prayer. Then bring your focus to your breath.

⫸ Listen to whatever presents itself. As thoughts arise, observe them and turn them around in your mind for a bit; then let them go. Again, bring the focus back to your breath.

⫸ Continue this practice, aware of the thoughts that grab your attention most strongly and quickly. Notice when you have been pulled away, and come back to the breath.

⫸ After a while, bring your focus directly to the stress at the heart of your prayer. Bring a gentle curiosity to it and see what it can teach you. Then let it go, like releasing a helium-filled balloon.

⫸ Sit in silence for a few minutes longer, as you observe the actions of mind, body, and spirit. When you feel ready, release and stretch.

Exploration: Mindful exhalation

Breathing is the bridge between our external and internal environments. Through respiration, the air around us is drawn deep inside our lungs, where it is processed and circulated before returning to the world outside. In a continuous flow, one breath is released to make space for another. In this natural cycle, the exhalation is linked to relaxation and the sense of well-being. It's understood in expressions such as, "breathing a sigh of relief" and "breathing easy."

The breath gives us constant feedback that reflects every aspect of our being. Let's continue our breathing exploration by observing the process of exhalation. With awareness, we can lengthen and cultivate its calming effect on our body, mind, and spirit. Follow the exhalation across the bridge, and enter a space of stillness deep inside. Here is a practice to help mindfully influence the breath.

Practice

⫸ Make yourself comfortable while sitting or lying down. Invite every part of yourself to relax as completely as possible. Give yourself a minute or two to observe this process. Notice any sensations of softening or letting go. Smile.

⫸ Begin to follow your breath. Observe how your breath moves through your body. Enjoy the movement. Gently bring your awareness to your belly. Watch it rise with the inhalation and fall with the exhalation. Can you feel the continuous wave-like movement of your breath deep inside?

» Without changing anything, bring your attention to the exhalation and to the sensations of letting go. Softly breathe in and breath out. Allow your awareness to glide down with the exhalation. Feel how your belly sinks back as the breath is released. Feel how your belly expands with each new breath.

» As you feel ready, very gradually lengthen the exhalation. Stay within your sense of comfort. Effortlessly, the exhalation relaxes every cell in your body. Return to your regular breathing pattern whenever you feel the need. Each breath is smooth and even. Enjoy the exhalation.

» At the bottom of the exhalation there is a space. Rest briefly in this space. Relax into the pause between breaths. Trust the inhalation. It will find its way to you. Receive the breath. Follow a long exhalation into the sacred space deep inside. You are safe and secure. Breathe in and out of this space, and allow it to expand. Be in this sanctuary. Be free to let go of anything. Release with the exhalation.

» Take your time. As you feel ready, come back to normal breathing. Slowly open your eyes. Move and stretch.

Reflections

As you become more familiar with extending the exhalation, try it with your eyes open. Mindful exhalation is a very practical tool. Its calming effect can relax the body, reduce anxiety, and soften hard feelings. You can practice it almost anywhere and anytime. Mini exhalation breaks are a great way to release the tension of a busy day. Be creative and leave practice reminders on your computer screen or scatter them throughout the kitchen. Lengthen the exhalation before a business meeting, school conference, or medical procedure. Follow the exhalation during an argument or when someone starts to push your buttons. Practice mindful exhalation at bedtime to promote more restful sleep.

With time, a mindful breathing practice begins to expand our emotional and psychological space.

Review

>> Stress is anything that applies tension in our lives and is a necessary part of life.

>> *Eustress* is perceived as positive and life-enhancing, whereas *distress* is perceived as life-depleting. Your body does not know the difference between the two.

>> Chronic, unrelenting distress can lead to illness and disease.

>> A method to manage stress can be remembered as PQRRS: **Practice** cultivating awareness so that we know stress when it affects us. **Question** our reactions or whatever comes up with gentle curiosity. **Reframe** situations from a more broad and compassionate perspective. **Respond** based on conscious choice, grounded in understanding and insight. **Surrender** any attachments to outcomes.

>> Stress management relies heavily on our point of view: What's eustress for one person may be distress to another.

>> Stress tends to flow in and through our relationships with ourselves, others, and the natural world.

>> Personality type can influence our reactions to stress in important, modifiable ways.

>> Physical activity can help manage stress.

>> There are many mind-focused tools that help relieve distress, including meditation, guided imagery, and breath-focused practice.

>> An approach to spirituality can help with reframing and surrendering.

Yoga Bits

>> Notice when you are reacting to stress and watch yourself without judging. How do you act, think, and feel in your body?

>> If you can catch yourself reacting to stress, take a single, conscious breath.

>> When something causes you distress, name it.

>» Lengthen your exhalation for several breaths at specific times throughout the day.

>» When you find yourself fixating on a specific stressor, actively release it for just one minute.

>» Close your eyes and visualize being in your favorite place in the world. Take four conscious breaths there, and return.

>» Take a moment to scan your body. If there is tension, breathe into it. If there is none, look for ways in which you can do less with your muscles while settling in to your current position.

STEP 7:
SPIRITUALITY

Spirituality exists wherever we struggle with the issue of how our lives fit into the greater cosmic scheme of things.... An idea or practice is "spiritual" when it reveals our personal desire to establish a felt-relationship with the deepest meanings or powers governing life.
—Robert C. Fuller

What is spirituality?

People define spirituality in many different ways. Some view it as a way to find peace, hope, and meaning in life, or as a way to praise and understand a Higher Power. Others see it as a way to follow a set of rules and rites defined by a specific religion, and still others believe spirituality is a particular experience or state of enlightenment. All of these definitions are valid.

Does spirituality mean attaining the highest stage of moral development, or is it a completely different kind of self-development that includes a broad focus on the universal qualities of beauty, creativity, and unconditional love? A great deal of work has been done to try to understand and define an optimal approach to spirituality. For our purposes, spirituality is the seat of the three-legged stool of health, supported by physical activity, stress management, and nutrition. All of these elements stand on awareness, and all aspects of our experiences influence them. Sound like a lot of variables? We'll try to make sense of this in a practical and sustainable way.

Spirituality and the three-legged stool of health

We can sense imbalances in our spiritual life when we apply the foundation of awareness. Every part of the three-legged stool is connected, and vital to its function. On the stool, spirituality and awareness are the only parallel elements. One could say that our spirituality reflects our awareness. If our awareness is cloudy and poorly developed, our spiritual view is limited. With broader awareness, we begin to see things as they are, and our spirituality becomes expansive.

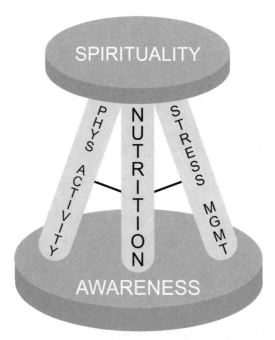

But we need to be careful here. Awareness can be very limited or it can be expansive, and we can incorrectly view our degree of awareness. We don't know what we don't know. It's possible to be very aware of a completely self-oriented view. As a result, spirituality will mirror that perception. In the name of a specific version of God, or country, or self-advancement, humans throughout history have managed to destroy each other, disregard views other than their own, and dismiss the natural world as a commodity to serve selfish needs. We can see this on a societal and global level, where people try to eradicate those unlike themselves, invade other countries, and create laws that shelter the rich and diminish the poor, all while thinking that they're following a spiritual path.

We can also see this on an individual level, where we dismiss in judgment what is too difficult to manage and we deny parts of ourselves. Oftentimes, we project these shadowy parts of ourselves onto others, giving us a reason to dismiss them as people as well. This doesn't paint a pretty picture. It reveals why cultivating awareness on our own, without questioning and support, can't be the sole answer. In short, we must recognize that spiritual growth and change can result in better spiritual health, and that there are higher and better levels.

For our purposes, we'll define **spiritual health** as finding internal and external balance with an individual's highest and final concern. This highest and final concern informs our thoughts and actions and gives meaning to all aspects of life, including all participants at all levels of their being and experience. Optimal spiritual health has a positive impact for the highest and best balance for the individual internally and for any other part of the whole system externally.

Throughout history, we see the fruits of higher levels of human interaction and associate these with higher stages of spiritual health. Clear awareness of a more inclusive, less self-focused worldview allows an inclusive spirituality and healing on all levels. We find this on a global level, where people volunteer their time, talents, and resources freely in the service of others, without any expectation of return. People support each other in times of crisis, create new ways to communicate, positively cultivate the natural world around them, and create social systems that protect basic human rights. On an individual level, one can embrace the process of healing, allowing a safe space for growth and change. Individuals can promote health and wholeness, and learn how to decrease suffering and increase enjoyment of life. You are doing just that through your life practice and by reading this book.

Religion and spirituality

Does one need to be involved in a specific religion in order to be spiritual? Can we be religious and not spiritual, or spiritual and not religious? Surveys have shown that about 25 percent of Americans consider themselves to be spiritual but not religious.[1] For our purposes, **religion** is a set of rules and rituals that are practiced and shared in a community. Religions include the major faith traditions of the world. **Spiritual** practices are those that intend to improve and nurture spiritual health, and aren't necessarily attached to a specific religious tradition. Spirituality and religion can exist both separately and together.

It's helpful to think about what barriers prevent the development of higher levels of spiritual health. Many individuals have lost the will to move forward spiritually because of unhealthy experiences with ungrounded spiritual practices or religious traditions. Many spiritual tools have been used outside of their cultural context and have lost some of the initial features that encouraged spiritual growth. Yoga and its commercialization is a good example: Originally, Yoga was intended as a balanced way to unite the mind, body, and spirit. Now, it's often approached as merely a type of physical activity. Many Yoga teachers and students are unaware of its spiritual aspects and potential power. As a consequence, the modern expression of Yoga can become unstable, if not unhealthy.

When discussing religious traditions, it's helpful to think about the word *faith*. In order to have faith in something, one must begin by not knowing. When we know that something is a fact, faith is no longer involved, and we move into the realm of knowledge. Faith requires surrendering to uncertainty and the unknown, whereas true knowledge requires understanding and insight. The two are not mutually exclusive, but when religion is out of balance, the lines can blur. Suddenly, faith becomes absolute knowledge of the correctness of a certain path. Knowledge limited to self-interest leads people to believe that the rules of that path apply to anyone and anything. These rules may then become something that followers believe are important enough to kill or die for.

On a less-severe level, a significant barrier to the success of religious traditions in nurturing spiritual health is a lack of more in-depth spiritual exploration beyond following simple rules and rituals. The container for deep spiritual work is created, but it's not nurtured in practice. Imagine solemnly praying in a church service only to have fellow churchgoers cut you off at the exit in a rush to go somewhere else. In sum, one of the main barriers to spiritual health is the focus on translation of rules, tools, and rituals, without any focus on transformation.

Due to the important nature of spirituality, our lack of discernment in identifying an optimal approach to it has historically resulted in massive problems. World wars have been fought over whose path to spirituality is the best, trying to force allegiance to a particular path or set of rules. Perhaps no other area of human experience has been associated with this level of historical disagreement.

This chapter is presented with humility and without assumptions. Remember that one of the basic tenets of our work here is creating a safe space. This safe space is a confidential holding of whatever comes up without trying to fix it. When an approach to spirituality is unbalanced, the Great Mystery that created and sustains the universe can somehow become a huge fixer-upper. It's especially important to avoid the temptation to judge each other in a heavy-handed fashion, or to pitch a spiritual or religious practice as an answer to another individual's difficulties. It's a good thing to share personal experiences or stories, and if someone is interested, he or she can ask for further resources.

Spiritual health

We can develop an optimal approach by looking at spiritual health the same way as other parts of our health. Just as we objectively determine what a higher level of physical fitness looks and feels like, we can define higher levels of spiritual health.

Spiritual health is viewed from two perspectives: the outside looking in and the inside looking out. Our integrative process will encourage both. The way we practice our spirituality has a major impact on others. Our goal is to develop an optimal and individual spiritual health practice that allows all participants the same opportunity to pursue sustainable wellness in their lives.

Spiritual stages

Spiritual stages can be thought of as the community in which we live, whereas **spiritual tools** are the ways we experience where we live—the different buildings, landscapes, and living areas. We stay at stages all of the time and we use tools occasionally. Whatever the stage, we see the world through the lens of that stage all of the time. The stage in which we operate will influence how we act from a mental, emotional, spiritual, social, political, and societal perspective. When we're visiting or using a particular tool, such as asking prayer, meditation, volunteering, practicing unconditional love, practicing forgiveness, experiencing a sense of oneness with all things, or feeling compassion for all living beings, we see the world through the lens of that tool for a little while, and then go to some other place in the community, or use some other tool to meet a need.

Distinct spiritual stages have a specific tendency to make use of certain spiritual tools because they match that stage's point of view, just as certain communities around the world tend to have defining characteristics. The particular tool we use may be more or less of a fit with the predominant stage through which we see the world. (See Table 7–1.) For example, a modern high-rise that looks normal in New York City may look out of place in Paris. As we grow in spiritual health, more tools become consistently available for use. This is just like physical health: The more physically fit one becomes, the more options are available to maintain internal and external balance.

Stage of Spiritual Health	Matching Tools
3: The All	Mystical religion, soul-mind-heart-body are one, being life, asking, listening, and acting prayer
2: The Other	Advanced religion, mind-body are one, doing life, some mind-heart-body connection, asking and listening prayer
1: The Self	Basic religion, physical emphasis, making it through life, some mind-body connection, asking prayer

Table 7–1: Stages of Spiritual Health and Matching Tools

Higher spiritual stages both transcend and include lower stages. A person living at a higher stage will not float away because he or she forgets to care for the self. He or she understands the lower stage completely and acts accordingly as the situation requires. Those operating at a lower stage may experience tools that bring insight into higher stages, but they don't fully understand or apply higher-stage perspective to their lives on a daily basis.

For our purpose, there are three spiritual stages defined by the individual's highest and final concern:

1. The Self
2. The Other
3. The All

Stage 1 is focused on the individual self and its needs. The main focus here is survival needs, such as food, water, and shelter. People in this stage are also focused on what they have to do in order to feel as though they are in control and able to protect their self-interests. The self can include whomever or whatever they see as the self—their group, community, team, culture, or whatever it is that meets their needs. They see the world literally and their main concern is physical. These individuals *make it through life* by using the body and the mind to get what they want. Spiritual tools in this stage are focused on asking for what will serve the needs of the self.

Stage 2 individuals see the world through the lens of self and also include the lens of others, and not just as a means to get what they want for themselves. The other and the self are seen as equally important. The world and all teachings can be seen literally but also from a moral and symbolic perspective, which contains opposites as a part of a whole. The heart, mind, and body work together to maintain internal and external balance. Individuals in Stage 2 mostly *do life* and can see things both literally and symbolically. Spiritual tools include asking for the needs of the self and others, and also making space for contemplative listening as a means of facilitating intuition, insights, and understanding.

Stage 3 individuals see the interplay of self and others while also including all living existence. These individuals think globally, even universally. For those living with The All as their ultimate concern, life has gone beyond the experience of the self and other as separate, into a life that transcends and includes all experience. Stage 3 individuals are able to *be life*. The soul, mind, heart, and body operate together as one. Their lives become a prayer. They can comfortably live with paradoxes through nondual thinking, whereby opposites are seen as different sides of the same coin. Fulfillment and despair simply cannot exist without each other, and the same can be said of light and darkness. Freed from the need to judge any temporary thought or feeling as good or bad, these individuals live in the eternal present moment.

An individual who operates at any of these stages can have experiences that include the use of temporary tools. We can choose to use specific tools that correspond with higher stages in order to exercise our spirit and encourage growth.

Let's follow an individual as he experiences these stages. At birth, we all start at Stage 1—focused on the self and our individual survival needs. Others are seen only as conduits for providing for those needs. We grow and change in ways that make our needs met both internally and externally as best as possible. Some individuals may stay at this stage permanently due to a variety of reasons—mainly having to do with the whole integrated world in which they live. If everyone this person comes into contact with is living at Stage 1, it's likely that this is where that individual will stay. If physical and basic needs are met poorly, it's also likely that these will become a high priority, and the individual will keep his focus in this stage. "Live and let die" is his mantra. Life and all of its teachings are seen literally, with clearly defined black-and-white answers. The needs of the self dominate all experience at whatever level.

But let's say that at some point this individual begins to experience situations in which his personal needs become less important. Let's say that he gets a glimpse of the fact that without sadness there would be no such thing as happiness. Let's say that his normal life leads him through challenges like great love or great suffering, which push his boundaries, and he is somehow initiated into a new way of seeing and being. Perhaps slowly, perhaps suddenly, he sees that the needs of the other are as important as the needs of the self. He will have entered Stage 2—The Other. "Live and let live" becomes his motto. It's possible and even preferable to live in such a way that the needs of The Other are not denied while satisfying the needs of The Self. The mind and body are seen as one and there is engagement with the heart of life. This heart of life drives decision making that is moral and allows the individual to explore his unique self. This stage sees him developing his talents in the service of self and others.

Stage 2 is where the individual may stay, especially if that is the dominant stage of all participants with whom he interacts. But let's say that some great suffering, teacher, or experience, such as losing something or someone held dear to him, comes along and brings with it a deep connection to a higher and final concern that includes everything. The individual transforms to Stage 3, now ultimately concerned about The Self, The Other, and The All. "Live and let's live together" becomes his mantra. The soul is fully encountered as the individual experience of the divine nature in all things. A relationship with this soul is nurtured, and the soul, mind, heart, and body act as one. Things can be seen from multiple perspectives—moral, literal, symbolic—and what can be called *both/and*, non-dual, or "not two."

Transforming and translating

All three stages of spiritual health are very broad brushstrokes, and there are shades of development that overlap along the way. The main point is that there are higher levels of spiritual health and these are attainable through a combination of diligent practice and compassion. We can firmly and gently direct our awareness to the evolution of a highest and final concern that includes all of life, all of existence.

We can apply the PQRRS practice to spirituality as well and ground our approach to spirituality in a daily *practice* of cultivating awareness. We *question* how our choices and actions define our highest and final concern. We *reframe* our possible choices and actions based on a larger perspective. We then *respond* in a way consistent with that larger perspective. Finally, we *surrender* our need to control the outcome, especially the need to be rewarded for good behavior as though spirituality was a sort of worthiness contest. The final step, surrender, is a vital approach to spirituality in which we can practice both non-striving and specific growth-oriented spiritual exercises at the same time.

Transition between stages is considered transformation, whereas using spiritual tools—such as contemplative prayer, volunteering, serving those in need, participating in ceremonies, practicing forgiveness and gratitude, healing old wounds, taking part in rituals, and offering our talents in the service of others—are translations. Spiritual transformation is the ultimate way that we see things with new eyes, or empty our cup. We can understand the stages and their implications with our intellect, but we don't transform to see the world at the level of that stage through intellect alone. Usually some form of lived experience brings us to transformation.

Purposeful lived experiences: Rituals and exercises

Healthy religious and cultural initiation rituals and spiritual exercises can guide us through transformational experiences. These approaches allow us to move to higher stages of spiritual awareness. They provide methods to develop a container, or safe space, for lived experience.

For example, Catholic children are led through the process of First Reconciliation, Holy Communion, and then Confirmation. These milestones are spaced over time. First Reconciliation teaches them the power of self-reflection and forgiveness. Holy Communion teaches that all Christians are connected and a part of the same body and bread of life. Confirmation requires a mature affirmation of spiritual practice, along with choosing a new name to acknowledge this transformation. Each of these processes allows for new and repeated experiences of growth beyond pure self-interest.

Native American cultures have Vision Quests and Sundance rituals that guide the initiate through various physical, mental, and emotional challenges in order to become a leader of their people. In a Vision Quest, the seeker goes through ritual fasting and then journeys alone to sacred areas. Here he or she prays and wait for visions that will direct his or her life's work. The Sundance ritual provides a visible connection between the natural world and the suffering of the people that the initiate must endure to be accepted as a potential leader. It does this through trials of physical endurance and pain.

The retreats and groups that we facilitate can be seen as a transformational-spiritual approach. We follow certain rituals, such as lighting a group candle and holding silence together. One key to the healthy use of rituals is to make sure that the tool does not become more important than the people involved. When this occurs, healthy ritual can become unhealthy superstition. For example, if we are holding silence together at a retreat and someone speaks, it does not mean that this person has committed an offense and must be reprimanded in some way. Healthy ritual creates a container in which spiritual experience can be held, and because spirituality is a powerful part of life, this container must be grounded in a merciful and non-judging awareness.

Richard Rohr, a Franciscan monk and founder of the Center for Action and Contemplation, has explored initiation rituals from around the world. In them, he found five major themes. He calls these *the five hard facts of life*. He also found five insights that come from the hard facts of life, which he calls *the five wonderfuls*.² It's important to note that healthy religion and initiation rituals do more than deliver these messages on a piece of paper for intellectual understanding, but actually facilitate realizations through lived experience.

The five hard facts of life are:

1. Life is hard.
2. You are not that important.
3. Your life is not about you.
4. You are not in control.
5. You are going to die.

The fact that life is hard is also one of the major tenets of Buddhism: Life is suffering. Clearly, life is not primarily about self-interests. Our powerlessness stimulates humility, trust, surrender, and patience. Death is a great equalizer and its inevitability helps us grow beyond pure self-interests. Our problems and disagreements are seen from a different perspective when we imagine their importance two hundred years in the future. Facing death makes life more precious as we learn to live with present-moment awareness.

Rohr's corresponding five wonderfuls are given mainly from a Christian perspective, and each refers to a biblical quote or event. They come out of the lived experience of initiation rituals.

1. "My yoke is easy and burden light." Life may be hard, but when lived in alignment with a higher power, the flow of life becomes smoother.
2. "Every hair on your head is counted." You see your individual self as limited, but at the level of the Great Mystery that is God, you are a valued and essential part of the grand plan.
3. Your life is not about you, but we all have been given specific talents and gifts from the Creator in order to serve ourselves and others.
4. You are not in control, but you do have free will. You can choose to respond in whatever way you discern is best and can move beyond purely self-oriented reactions to more informed choices that benefit all participants involved.
5. You are going to die, but resurrection is a fact. You can see this clearly by observing the life cycles of nature. The spring flowers appear to wither and die in the winter, only to return again.

Moving forward

It's essential to move through spiritual development with discipline and compassion, firmly and gently recognizing the needs of ourselves and others. It's important to acknowledge that awareness grounds our efforts. Anywhere along the way is a wonderful place to be. There is potential for growth and change, no matter where we are. Non-attachment, letting go, surrender, and non-judgment are all vital to moving forward as we continuously empty and fill our cup.

How will you know when you are moving along the path in a positive direction? Using the garden analogy, when we water seeds of forgiveness, mercy, awareness, and love, their fruits speak for themselves. These fruits increase the ability to enjoy life while being patient and kind with ourselves and others. Nothing can eliminate pain, but spiritual practice can help us to reframe it so that we respond with compassion and understanding, rather than resistance and suffering. With this continuum in mind, let's explore an integrative approach to spirituality.

Spirituality and all participants

A community in which to practice is one of the key ingredients to a sustainable approach. The greater number of people that practice together, the more impact the work will have. A group is generally more effective than a single person at decreasing the suffering of others and improving their enjoyment of life.

Questions to ponder:

- » How does our spiritual practice influence others in our family, community, society, and throughout the world?
- » How do these levels of relationships influence our practice?
- » What are the greatest issues that create inequalities in your world today?
- » Are these issues social, political, economic, or service-related?
- » What small action can you take to address these issues?

Spirituality and the natural world

The natural world is a major resource for spiritual practice. Just observing nature can have a calming effect. We can hold in mind our highest and final concern in life and see how it aligns with what we observe in nature while resting in a quiet, natural environment. The vast beauty of the natural world and its inherent spirituality can fill us with wonder and bring a sense of peace.

Try the following exercise wherever you meet the natural world:

≫ Find a safe and quiet place outside. It could be a spot in your backyard, in a park, at the beach, in the mountains, or on the balcony of your apartment building.

≫ Whether you're on a bench, in a chair, or sitting or lying directly on the ground, exhale and consciously release the weight of the body as completely as possible. Let go of anything you'd like to let go of, physically, mentally, or emotionally. Return to the Earth what no longer serves you. Invite every muscle to relax. Allow your lips to soften into a slight smile and relax your eyes. Follow the breath as it flows through your body. Observe the physical sensations of breathing. When the thinking mind pulls you away, gently return to the feeling experience.

≫ Bring awareness to the natural world around you. Observe the rhythms of nature through your senses. Hear the sounds of creatures all around you. Just listen. Feel the warmth of the sun or the cool of the air against your skin. Just feel. See the colors and shapes of plants and trees. Just see. Smell the scents of animals and earth. Just smell.

≫ Be curious and receptive. Allow your awareness to settle on a single sensation—the song of a bird, the scent of a flower, the movement of tree branches in the wind. Give steady focus to whatever you're most attuned. Imagine having this experience for the first time, unconnected to any other. Absorb the nature of it. Align with the spirit of it. Lovingly give your attention to its every aspect. Be here, moment by moment.

≫ As you feel ready, gently release the object of focus. Bring your awareness back to the breath. Slowly move and stretch. Notice how you feel.

Our actions affect the natural world. If our highest and final concern is purely focused on ourselves, we may come to see the natural world as only something to meet our individual needs.

Questions to ponder:

≫ How can we practice caring for the natural world so that it will be there for our children's grandchildren?

≫ What are the biggest issues that threaten the natural world?

≫ How can we be a part of the solution?

Spirituality and culture

Specific cultures have different ways of looking at the world and different highest and final concerns. We can think about the predominant spiritual stage of health in a culture. Is your culture in the Self, Other, or All stage of spiritual health? How does that influence your thoughts and actions?

Freedom of religious practice is one of the founding principles of the United States Constitution and also the Universal Declaration of Human Rights. How do we balance our religious or spiritual practice with those who choose other practices?

Spirituality and the lens of self

The Enneagram personality types help us understand our basic desires and fears. They ultimately tell us about our strengths and weaknesses. Our personalities are expressed differently depending on our stage of spiritual health. At the self-oriented stage, we will express our weaknesses more often than we would if we were living in the other-oriented stage. The Enneagram can help us catch ourselves in the act of making knee-jerk reactions. This practice alone can help us become more spiritually healthy.

What do our personalities have to do with finding internal and external balance with our highest and final concern? We can think of our best self-expression as one that has resolved the issues presented by basic fears and desires. Our ultimate concern becomes less self-oriented by definition. Our internal resources are freed from a self-preservation focus and brought to how our unique gifts and talents can best flow with the process of life.

Some would call this process a movement from the limited, self-oriented, and false self to the expansive, authentic, and connected true self.

Bringing our focused awareness to our interactions with all situations in life can be an important learning tool. We initially become aware of *who we think we are* by watching our automatic reactions, and gradually live *who we really are* based on our conscious choices. In this light, everything becomes our teacher.

Spirituality and the body

Many spiritual tools work to bring the spirit's expression into physical form. When the body is viewed as a temple, caring for it becomes a form of spiritual practice. A balanced Yoga practice supports embodied spirit in rhythm with the natural world.

The body is the felt experience of all that is material in this world. The word *Christ* is seen by some to denote the ultimate balance of the spiritual and material. We neither deny the material world to focus only on the spiritual nor totally immerse ourselves in the spiritual world while ignoring the physical. Balancing the spiritual and material takes effort, but it's key to a sustainable approach on all levels.

Questions to ponder:

» How do you balance the spiritual and material sides of yourself?

» Can you think of a time when you were out of balance in this regard? How did it feel?

» What can you do to maintain your balance moving forward?

The following exercise is a helpful meditation that links spirituality with physical movement. We'll first describe the movement and then give the words to be repeated silently or aloud. Figures are shown to help you follow the movements.

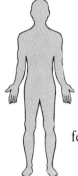

Exercise: The tree of life

Begin standing with your feet a comfortable distance apart and your arms at your sides. Give the weight of your body to the ground, and allow yourself to be supported. Imagine growing roots from the back of your pelvis, down through your legs and ankles, and from the soles of your feet. These roots reach deeply into the earth.

Place your hands over your heart. Rest here for a breath or two and follow the gentle movements of your breath. Feel the connection to all Nature through your body. Say silently or aloud: "Rooted in Nature."

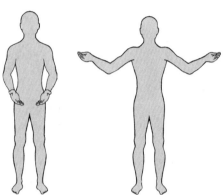

Move your hands and arms out from your heart and open yourself to Spirit. Extend your arms out to the side like the growing branches of a tree reaching out into the world around you. Say silently or aloud: "Open to Spirit."

Slowly move both of your arms to the left. Return to center with arms reaching in opposite directions. Slowly move both arms to the right. Again, return to center. Imagine expanding your life experience in all directions. Say silently or aloud: "Expanding."

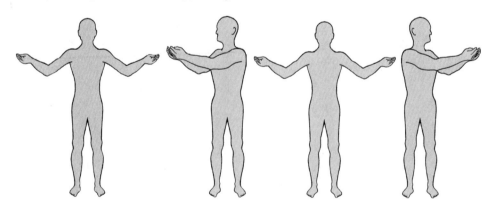

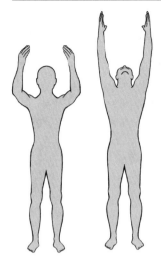

Rooted in awareness, slowly extend your arms toward the sky. Stretch your arms up as far as you are comfortable. Like the Tree of Life, you are the link between heaven and earth. Say silently or aloud: "In awareness."

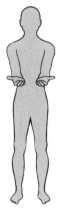

Slowly lower your arms in front of you until they are nearly waist high, with palms facing up. Imagine the energy of all Creation raining down on you and filling you with wisdom and strength. Say silently or aloud: "I am filled."

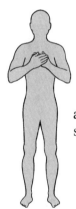

Bring your hands back to your heart. Follow the movement of your breath. Feel the connection with heaven above and the earth below. Say silently or aloud: "With wisdom and strength."

Release your arms and slowly reach toward the ground, perhaps bending at your knees and waist to touch the ground. Offer nourishment to the Tree of Life. Say silently or aloud: "Through the Tree of Life."

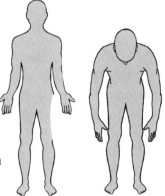
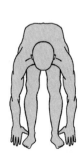

Slowly come back to standing. With palms together, bring your hands to your heart. Honor the place where Spirit dwells, in the space where there is only one. Say silently or aloud: "Namaste." (See page 204 for a discussion of *Namaste*.)

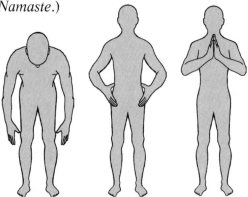

This exercise focuses our intention on bringing a new balance to the spiritual and material world. The word *grace* is often used to describe something we've received from a Higher Power without it being a reward for performance of any kind. Another way to think of grace is that it brings what's currently not in existence into a place where it can be experienced. Grace brings the unknown into the known. This exercise is grace in action. It brings an unknown balance of the spiritual and material into a visible exercise and known intention.

Spirituality and the mind

Franciscan monk and author Richard Rohr wisely said, "If you do not transform your pain, you are destined to transmit it." The mind can be either a significant assistant or an impediment to spiritual health. We'll focus on the power of forgiveness and love, while releasing judgment of ourselves and others. We'll bring our awareness to the way that we put up barriers to the natural expression of our highest self.

Giving or denying forgiveness is one of the clearest ways this can happen. When Jesus taught his students how to pray, one of the key messages was: "Forgive our trespasses as we forgive those who have trespassed against us." When we forgive, we are forgiven. What we choose to remember about any situation is central to this process. Forgiveness is a powerful spiritual tool and a way to approach unity for ourselves and others.

There is a significant interplay among our abilities to forgive, judge, and empathize. The following story is an amalgamation of several tales told by wise mentors to an audience of students:

When I was a child, there was one person who rode on the bus with us to and from school that no one wanted to sit beside. As a matter of fact, no one wanted to interact with this boy at all. He smelled bad, wore dirty clothes, and wasn't nice to others. He was seen as the school bully, and no one wanted to cross his path. One day on the way home, the bus had to take a different route because of an accident. Instead of dropping me off first, the driver pulled through a part of town that I had never seen before. The bus slowed in front of a particularly old and run-down house. There were broken bottles in the lawn and trash all around. Some of the windows were broken, with cardboard filling in the gaps. There was an older adult sitting on the porch with a bottle of alcohol by his side. The boy that nobody wanted to be near walked forward from his seat in the back and stepped out of the bus. I then realized that maybe if I lived in the same situation as this boy, perhaps I would be just like him. I realized that when we know the whole story, judgment usually turns to compassion.

There's almost always more to a story than meets the eye, especially when most of the time we're thinking about how to meet our own needs—this holds back both the other individual and ourselves. Understanding of the whole situation usually brings about new insight. Even if we never have the opportunity to see the whole picture from the other person's perspective, even if we never receive the grace of our perception taking a detour around life as usual, we can give one another the benefit of the doubt.

When we allow ourselves the opportunity to see things from a new perspective, we become open to transformation—to letting go of the old. Old pains can often be perceived as coming from outside of ourselves. On deeper reflection, they often tap into what we might call the shadow side of ourselves. This shadow side is usually a part of ourselves that we can't accept and is related to our deepest fear.

Working with our shadow side

Our shadow side is neither good nor bad. For example, think of life as a large park filled with well-spaced trees. Some of the trees are smaller and some are larger than others. The trees represent all of the ideas, lessons, personality traits, and concepts that have been programmed into our life. The sun above shines light on these trees, helping them grow. They define the park of our life. Beneath these trees, there is shadow. We tend to spend most of our lives in the light and expressing what we have learned. We catch glimpses of our shadow as it's represented in the thoughts, ideas, or people outside of us. For example, someone who is taught to "never do anything half-baked" will be very diligent. The shadow of this statement makes it difficult for this person to let go and be free-spirited. When she encounters people, thoughts, or ideas expressing a free-spirited and "let go" approach to life, the diligent person may become frustrated.

Our shadow presents an opportunity to learn from a *both/and* perspective and include all of our self while broadening our range of possible responses. For the shadow-side example, it may be an option for the diligent individual to do things in a totally committed fashion but also be free spirited as the situation dictates. It's helpful to inquire: If I were born and raised under different circumstances, would I have acted in the same way as the person, thought, or idea that I find distasteful? Once we get beyond our immediate reaction of one thing as right and the other wrong, we can hold open a space to discern the value of a person, thought, or idea based on more than just our personal bias.

We generally fear dark spaces because of the unknown. But when we acknowledge the fearful and shadowy parts of ourselves, we can give them love. Love brings the mind and heart together. Love can seem like a four-letter word to be avoided in polite conversation, or it can seem like an unattainable ideal. Love is really a simple and natural thing that we all do, give, and come into contact with. There is a *doing* part of love and a *being* part. The doing part is when we apply our desire to relieve suffering and increase enjoyment of life, either for ourselves or for another. We don't want ourselves or others to hurt. This active part of love that addresses the pain of others is called compassion. We want ourselves and others to be happy, and we act with kindness in order to make this happen. Unconditional love is a powerful force that fills our being so that we can give love in the service of self and others. As St. Thomas Aquinas said, love allows us "to will the good of another."

The being part of love is when we seek unity with our whole self or with another. Perhaps one of the reasons that our defenses can go up when we hear the word *love* is associated with this being-oriented use of the word. Love as unification can easily be misconstrued and potentially unhealthy for one party or the other. For example, a tiger could really love an antelope and want to become one with it totally. If the tiger consumes the antelope, that would be good for the tiger, but not good for the antelope. Love as being includes unity while honoring each individual's integrity. Love is *both/and*, not *either/or*. Love as being is without conditions and has no borders. It opens a space for acceptance that reaches beyond our basic fears and desires. It does not require that we are the same just because we are united.

Often we project onto others the very qualities we reject in ourselves. Mindful recognition of this tendency creates an opportunity for self-acceptance. Loving our judgmental and scared self can decrease our suffering and the suffering of others. Love does not try to eliminate or change our shadow side as a quick fix. It's a part of who we are, and it's neither positive nor negative. We may or may not like it at first, but we can become aware of it, love it, learn from it, and see it as a teacher. Experiencing love can lead to transformation. When we begin to look at our life experience with merciful awareness, we no longer pass suffering or unresolved pain on to others in the form of projection.

Here are some helpful exercises for working with your shadow:

Writing

Think about someone who either really annoys you or really inspires you. What about that individual is most annoying or inspiring? In one sentence, sum up what affects you the most about this individual. Now think about your own choices and actions. Summarize the pertinent ones in a sentence. How does your sentence align with the other individual's? Are there lessons, ideas, ideals, or experiences in your life that influence you to think, feel, and act in a certain way that relates to the annoying or inspiring aspect of the other individual?

Picture-drawing

The unconscious mind works using symbols. Symbols are images that represent something to the person using them. A door could represent a new beginning or a part of life that is closed off. The nature of symbols is non-dual. The door could represent both a closing and an opening. Symbols help us to see that opposites are really just different sides of the same coin, and one could not exist without the other. Picture-drawing is a good way to look at the light and dark sides of ourselves. Symbols are a way to communicate without having the filter of language get in the way of our expression. In our culture, we've developed a kind of conspiracy of superficial niceness. "How are you? Fine. How are you? Fine." Symbols get around this superficiality.

You don't need to be a great artist to do this exercise well. You'll need three blank, white pieces of paper and some crayons. Take a few moments to consider the following three questions:

1. What holds me back in life?
2. What supports me in life?
3. What does my ideal life look like?

Then focus on your breath for a few moments, and picture in your mind's eye that you are sitting in a dark movie theater. The curtain rises and a blank white screen fills your field of view. One by one, think about each question and wait for an image to appear in front of you on the screen that answers it. Don't try to process whatever comes up. Witness it with a gentle curiosity. Once you have an image in mind for each question, bring your focus back to the breath and then open your eyes and draw what you saw.

Use one single piece of paper for each question. Once you are done, you can share them in your group. Together, try to discuss the following:

» What is present on the sheet of paper?
» What is missing?
» What do these images mean to you?
» If the picture told a story, what title would you give each individual sheet?
» When you put all three together, what title would you give?

Once you have presented your picture, it may be helpful to hear how others would feel about the drawings if they had drawn them. If you are working in a group of people with similar life experience, this exercise can be very fruitful. When working on your own, it may be helpful to ask a loved one to look at the pictures with you.

Picture-drawing can be an incredibly beneficial way to gain insight from a part of ourselves that we don't usually access or communicate with. Dr. Matt used picture-drawing to select his medical specialty with the guidance of Dr. Bernie Siegel. Amazing details presented themselves, including an image depicting how many children he would have and his work facilitating groups.

Spirituality and the spirit

Is there a guiding force that creates all things or a universal intelligence that animates all of life? The way we answer the question has a tremendous effect on the way we see ourselves. If we see God as a gray-bearded and benevolent king sitting on a throne, our own personal self-image may be one of an obedient servant. If we recognize the Great Mystery giving life to all things, we may see our self as an integral part of that Mystery. Or we may believe that life is universal intelligence itself, and there is no supreme being. In this case, we may see ourselves as a part of an interdependent web of life. There is no right or wrong answer here. It's interesting to consider how our experience of whatever we call Spirit influences who we are and how we choose to act. Our image of Spirit creates our image of our self.

Questions to ponder:

» How do we expand our awareness beyond the ordinary?

» Does everything happen for a reason?

» How do you express spirituality?

» Can spirituality be measured and recognized?

» What is inner peace? What is enlightenment?

Our spiritual practice can focus on tools that facilitate a variety of experiences. We can consider our spiritual practice like a prayer. The kind of prayer we use depends on where we are on our spiritual journey.

As we advance through the stages of spiritual health, our focus expands. We begin with the internal experience of the Spirit that we can call the soul. Then we expand our focus and realize that there are many souls within one shared spirit. We then bring all of creation into view, acting as both a part of and the complete spectrum of a mature, evolving universe full of life.

As we move along the path and water the seeds of spiritual health, the fruits of our focus will emerge. Awareness allows us to choose love, joy, peace, patience, kindness, goodness, faithfulness, gentleness, and self-control. There is no perfect, unchanging state of spiritual balance. By bringing awareness to our spiritual health, we can grow and change. Our pain is transformed and creates the fertile soil from which spiritual fruits arise.

The word *Namaste* comes from ancient Sanskrit and generally means "I honor you." Used in India as a greeting and farewell, it has found its way into many American Yoga classes. The word is linked to a prayerful gesture, in which the hands are pressed together over the heart with the palms touching and the fingers pointed upward. Completed with a slight bow, the posture humbly recognizes and honors the place where the individual spirit dwells. *Namaste* unites us and symbolizes our spiritual interconnection. We offer this gesture to each other as a group in every Sustainable Wellness session, with these words:

Namaste. I honor the place in you where, when you are in that place in you, and I am in that place in me, there is only one of us.

Exploration: Mindful searching

In the spiritual sense, a search involves seeking something of deep meaning that's concealed or invisible to the eye. Its discovery requires expanded awareness and an inner journey that may take a lifetime. The lessons learned along the way can become tools for personal growth.

Our sophisticated computer technology allows us to search for a word or document within seconds. We can "Google" virtually anything, anytime. Type a few associated words and instant answers appear. Complex questions are answered effortlessly with a few keystrokes. We lose patience with slow computers. Our lives become organized around Internet connections.

Questions to ponder:

- » What happens to our spiritual connections in the process?
- » When does information become a burden?
- » Does our spirituality recede as external facts overpower internal knowing?
- » Will we lose the ability to consider open-ended questions?
- » Will we lose the ability to ponder the unanswerable?

Practice

Try the following practice to develop and explore a sense of space and openness. Can you sit with it?

1. Sit down straight with awareness. Establish a steady, comfortable posture. Gently close your eyes.
2. Give yourself permission to relax and soften. Begin to follow the breath.
3. There is nowhere to go and nothing to do. Be here breath-by-breath. Rest in the pause between breaths. Relax into the space between breaths and allow the space to expand.
4. Imagine a vast space all around you.
5. Imagine the infinite space inside you.
6. Relax. Breathe. Experience your body as a space within space.
7. Calm. Peaceful. Be here moment by moment. Contained by the unknowable. Be in this space without needing to fill it.
8. As you feel ready, very gently open your eyes.
9. Pay attention to how you feel.

Review

» Spiritual health is finding internal and external balance with an individual's highest and final concern.

» Religion and spirituality are not the same and are also not mutually exclusive.

» Spiritual stages advance from a focus on the Self to a focus on the Self and Other, to a focus that includes the Self, Other, and All of life.

» We can apply the PQRRS system to spirituality through awareness practice, questioning our actions and reactions, reframing our experience to include a broader view, responding with that broader view in mind, and then surrendering our attachment to outcomes.

» Transformation is key to moving to higher spiritual stages and improved spiritual health. It includes letting go of the old, or emptying the cup. Healthy rituals and exercises can lay the foundation for transformation and help us to grow and develop spiritually.

» We can recognize that we are moving on the right path spiritually when the fruits of our practice include an increased ability to enjoy life while being patient and kind with self and others. Forgiveness, gratitude, non-judgment, humility, patience, love, and kindness are also fruits of spiritual work.

» A sustainable spiritual approach includes a balance between the spiritual and material worlds.

» The shadow side of our self is neither good nor bad. It is merely an outcome of our innate gifts and life experiences. Working with shadow can increase self-understanding and broaden our range of possibilities.

» All spiritual tools can be thought of as a form of prayer. Some prayer includes asking, whereas other forms are focused on listening.

Yoga Bits

» Find quiet time each day—even if it's only in one-minute spaces.

» Spend time alone in nature even if just for a few conscious breaths.

» Listen to music that moves you.

» Read a poem, inspirational quote, or story each day.

» Practice contemplative prayer by just sitting and listening.

» Volunteer for a worthy cause.

» Be grateful for small things. Begin each day with thanks for three specific gifts in your life.

» Keep a journal of your thoughts, questions, and insights. Keep this handy throughout the day so you can easily record new insights and also revisit old ones when you're feeling overwhelmed.

» Express yourself through writing or drawing.

» Find something each day for which you can forgive yourself and others.

STEP 8:
BRINGING IT ALL TOGETHER

Efficiency is doing things right; effectiveness is doing the right things.
—Peter F. Drucker

How to begin

S mall drops of change flow into the river of life. Reshaping through time, the river meets storms and obstacles with greater fluency. Inexplicably, it moves forward by yielding to the present, while converging natural elements uncover hidden grooves. Like the river, we can move through life with mindful awareness to meet challenges, negotiate our tendencies, and sustain a larger view of life.

The previous chapters have offered many opportunities to explore an integrative approach to sustainable wellness. It begins with cultivating the ground of awareness that allows us to see the imbalances in life that affect nutrition, physical activity, stress management, and spirituality. Once identified, we can determine how and why an imbalance influences us. With practice, we learn to trace its roots and open a space to respond to events instead of reacting unconsciously. Life is witnessed through the many aspects of the individual self, including our dominant personality type and its basic fear and desire, vice and virtue. We see how previous life experiences impact every situation and influence future hopes.

Looking at situations as they affect us on all levels allows us to move forward. We can see how they influence, and are influenced by, all participants in the process, including the natural world. All the elements of a fully integrated life become allies and provide a larger perspective in which to reframe the imbalances that are sure to occur. Ultimately, this process allows us to make the best life choices for the highest good. Present-moment awareness frees us from dwelling on the past and anticipating the future. Moment by moment, we enter the flow of life to experience its unique unfolding.

New tools

You've experimented with many new tools throughout this book. All of these, in various combinations, have the potential to promote sustainable wellness in your life. How do you move forward now to bring these puzzle pieces together? How do you choose the most effective personal strategies and implement them efficiently throughout your life?

We recommend that you start small and let your life practice grow organically. Always begin with a deep understanding that there's nothing wrong with you. You can grow through change and remain content with who you are right now. These are not mutually exclusive states; they are different sides of the same coin. You're okay and there is room to grow. You will face many obstacles in coming to this realization. Some of the most common obstacles exist only as a product of the mind. We can learn to recognize a few patterns or families of thought that often show up. Naming these thoughts softens their effect and opens the door to questioning, reframing, and conscious choice. Here are some patterns of thought to look out for:

1. The never-enoughs: This family of thought leads us to believe that everything in life is in short supply. There is never enough for everyone to be content. As an individual, you are never enough just as you are. Acceptance, non-judging, non-striving, and beginning again help to hold the "never-enoughs" at bay.

2. The shoulda-coulda-wouldas: This group keeps us rooted in the past with thinking about what we should or could have done. It keeps us thinking that different choices concerning past actions

could have created a magically better outcome. Surrender is an especially potent antidote to this family of thinking.

3. The if-onlys: Close relatives to the shoulda-coulda-wouldas, this family finds the present moment deficient and believes that it could be better if only XYZ happened, so-and-so was present, and so on. The grass is always greener for the choice we didn't make. Patience, trust, and surrender help keep the "if-onlys" at arm's length.

In order to sustain your ability to grow and change, you need a tried and true method of emptying your cup, letting go of the old, and embracing new tools. Cultivating awareness on all levels is key to transformation and letting go. Consistently remaining open to the possibility of transformation brings freshness to life. With the ground of awareness firmly beneath the three-legged stool of health, an integrative approach helps you choose the proper tools.

An integrative planning process

When you begin to address an imbalance, ask yourself why the imbalance exists in the first place. The answer will help you better understand how to nurture yourself. At the same time, consider its impact on you and all of the participants in your life. The following checklist may be helpful. Make sure to stop, calm, and rest before beginning this exercise.

Exercise

1. I'm aware that I'm out of balance in the _____ part of my three-legged stool of health.

2. This imbalance may have roots in several parts of my life. I'll take a moment to think about each of the following areas and how they might contribute to this imbalance:
    a. My personality
    b. My past experiences
    c. My future plans
    d. My body
    e. My mind
    f. My spirit

g. All of the players involved

h. My culture

i. The natural world

3. Understanding the roots of the imbalance, I'll hold it in my awareness, waiting for insight and the ability to see things from a new perspective.

4. With insight, I'll develop an action plan to restore my balance in this particular area.

5. I'll embrace the new tool of _____. As I make this small change, I'll surrender to the process and check my progress often to see how it affects my balance.

6. I'll practice greater awareness in my life and meet any future imbalance with new eyes.

Developing a life practice

There are many ways to respond to small imbalances and uncover present-moment awareness throughout the day. Yoga Bits give us many simple options. At the same time, it's helpful to devise a broader plan that works on all levels of being and experience, with all participants in the process. Choose a specific tool that appeals to you and use Table 8–1 as a template to address imbalances from a mind-body-spirit perspective. Develop a broader plan and drop in the tool(s) at the appropriate time to rediscover balance. For instance, if your physical activity level is out of balance, you might try to exercise outdoors, with others, or in another way that fits your personality type.

Awareness, planning, action, maintenance, repeat

Remember this process from the beginning of our journey? This is the continuous cycle necessary for sustainability. Transformation is the fuel that charges the process. Focus on your desire to regain balance. Let your passion for life bring you into a full embrace with your true self at its highest and best. All of us experience struggles and failures, but when we live life with merciful awareness, obstacles and setbacks become teachers that guide us along the way.

	Self	Culture (including all participants, family, community, society)	Natural World
Body	10 minutes of planned physical activity that fits your personality type or exercise style	Participate in a planned activity with at least one other person	Take a walk in the woods
Mind	10 minutes of focus on your greatest desire in life	Take time to mindfully listen to another person without interrupting him or her	Enjoy the company of a companion animal for 10 minutes
Spirit	Shadow work—10 minutes of focus on a part of yourself that you find annoying when you see it in others	Volunteer your time in a way that reflects your highest and ultimate concern	Sit in nature and hold a troubling life issue in mind; listen for an answer

Table 8–1. Some Integrative Life Practice Options

The value of retreats

It's helpful to put aside some time every day for a health practice that focuses on your specific tools. Usually it takes time and persistence to empty your cup. Also, we've found it's very useful to have a period of time dedicated completely to caring for yourself—to go on retreat. The word *retreat* comes from the Latin word *retrahere*, meaning "to pull back." When we pull back from the busyness of our lives, we can see things from a new perspective. Consistently, we've witnessed the tremendous benefit of half-day, full-day, and week-long retreats.

In our experience, there are several essential elements necessary for a successful retreat. The first is letting go of any outcomes. It's impossible to know in advance what success will look like. As facilitators, we're well aware that we don't have the answers. Some of life's most important questions aren't riddles to be solved, but rather mysteries to be held softly. As we design retreat schedules, we can't be sure which, if any, tools or exercises may facilitate personal transformation. There is no way to transform another person. A retreat experience will look different for everyone, in every group.

Safe space is the foundation for our transformational retreats. This maintains a confidential holding, without judgment, of whatever comes up. It's also helpful to share this space with people who have similar experiences, especially if that experience is life-defining in some way. A situation is life-defining if it causes either great love or great suffering. People who share life-defining experiences develop a common language others may not comprehend.

The simple act of openly sharing stories, thoughts, worries, joys, and obstacles makes a safe space sacred. This may sound simple, but it's usually not easy. Remember: The work of healing involves paying attention with a merciful awareness to those parts of our life we would rather not look at. When we stop, calm, and rest, it may take some time for these long-neglected parts of our self to bubble up to the surface.

A general schedule for our retreats is offered in the Resources section as a guideline for your consideration (page 223). You may wish to hire massage therapists, chefs, creative arts therapists, Yoga instructors, or others to lead specific sessions or to deliver their service during the retreat. Every provider must be screened beforehand and understand the safe and sacred space into which they enter. If you are facilitating the retreat, or are in charge of finding care providers, we suggest you familiarize yourself with their work prior to the retreat. If the provider is going to cook, eat their food. If they are going to provide creative art therapy, do a project with them. And yes, if they are giving massages, experience a session with them (there are some perks to locating providers for a retreat!). Most importantly, there needs to be a match with the provider and this type of transformational work in a safe space.

Certain people have a knack for facilitating small groups. They're able to open a safe space and keep the group dynamics flowing along, moving the process through its necessary up and down cycles, similar to the in and out breaths. A facilitator should walk the talk and be open to exploring possibility and surrender. Many licensed clinical social workers are excellent group facilitators, though special training is not necessary. We have included a brief guide for facilitators in the Resources section on page 225. This guide for facilitators can also be helpful in maintaining your own health practice.

If you're working alone, you can develop your own retreat schedule based on these same resources and tools. We like to use tools that promote communication on all levels of being and experience. We try to cultivate mind, body, and spiritual connection in as many ways as possible.

The power of connection

As we've seen with our integrative model, we receive a great deal of energy and inspiration from working with a group. Once you've completed your eight weeks together, find a way to stay in touch. This adds another layer to the maintenance part of sustaining change. You could schedule quarterly meetings, or register your group at *www.sustainablewellnessonline.com* and join our ongoing community. You'll find resources for further practice on this site as well. The relationship you've formed with your group is a powerful one grounded in awareness and a safe, sacred space. After going through this experience with many groups, we've come to understand the subtle difference between questioning and inquiry. With questioning, we expect an answer. With inquiry, we pose a question without needing to know the answer. We welcome you to our ongoing community of inquiry, where part of sustainability is the ability to wonder together.

A new beginning

We offer here a poem that reflects our view of transformation and emptying the cup. Our entire life is like the cup that fills and empties; we let go and begin again. As we use the cup of our life, we can learn from the scratches, chips, and stains. Most of all, we can use what we have been given. When a group member first presented this poem, someone had changed the title to "The Chipped Cup." This is a commentary on where we choose to focus our awareness: on our defects instead of our inherent wholeness. Ours is a sustainable process that reminds us that a chipped cup is a perfect cup; a lived life, the perfect life.

"The Perfect Cup"
by Joyce Rupp

It is time for me to see the flaws of myself
and stop being alarmed

It is time for me to halt my drive
for perfection and to accept my blemishes

It is time for me to receive slowly evolving growth
the kind that comes in God's own good time
and pays no heed to my panicky pushing

It is time for me to embrace my humanness
To love my incompleteness

It is time for me to cherish the unwanted
to welcome the unknown
to treasure the unfulfilled

If I wait to be perfect before I love myself
I will always be unsatisfied and ungrateful

If I wait until all the flaws, chips, and cracks disappear
I will be the cup that stands on the shelf and is never used.

Take time to review your journey with us and trace the path you followed through the book. As you make practical steps to develop a daily health practice, refer to any written materials you produced, pictures you drew, and your journal or consumption diary, and pay attention to whatever comes up during the day. Review the practices, explorations, and Yoga Bits you feel most drawn to. Come back to the self-reflections exercise and life review. Consider changes you notice in the way you eat, move, manage stress, and relate to the world around you. Remember to ask yourself: How do I feel? What am I aware of? Where am I?

We suggest dedicating quiet time, even a few minutes here and there, to continue your exploration of breath and awareness. As frequently as you can, find a space to observe the river of life. Spread out the blanket of awareness. Give the weight of the body, mind, and emotions to the Earth below. Allow yourself to be supported. Follow the miracle of breath as it nourishes and inspires you. Return to the big sky of the mind, the sacred container that gently holds everything. Rest in the sky and release the ever-changing clouds of thought that pull you away from the eternal present. Surrender judgments and expectations. Enter the silence—the stillness where there is only one. Be here. Just be.

Yoga Bits

- ❧ Sit in a different place in your house or yard and gain a different perspective.
- ❧ Focus on your breath when stopped at a red light.
- ❧ Each time you log in to your computer at work, practice relaxing breath or do five seconds of neck rolls.
- ❧ When you wake up, think of one thing you are thankful for.
- ❧ When you go to sleep at night, review your day from start to finish and remember something that surprised you, something that inspired you, and something that moved you emotionally.

- » Establish a cue that happens often during the day. It could be a phone ringing or a specific sound, like a clock marking the hour. Each time you're cued, mindfully breathe in and breathe out for one breath before resuming your activity.

- » Think of something in your life that feels out of your control. Actively surrender your concern about it with an extended out breath or sigh, like filling a balloon and letting it float away.

- » When outdoors, notice a particular feature of the weather, sky, or landscape, and watch its activity without trying to figure it out.

- » Ask yourself "Where am I?" until the answer is "Here and Now."

Notes

Introduction

1. Eisenberg, D.M., R.C. Kessler, C. Foster, F.E. Norlock, D.R. Calkins, and T.L. Delbanco. "Unconventional Medicine in the United States: Prevalence, Costs, and Patterns of Use." *New England Journal of Medicine* 328.4 (January 28, 1993): 246–252.

2. Tan, S.Y., and P. Uyehara. "William Osler (1849–1919): Medical Educator and Humanist." *Singapore Medical Journal* 50.11 (November 2009): 1048–1049.

3. Ornish, D., G. Weidner, W.R. Fair, R. Marlin, E.B. Pettengill, C.J. Raisin, S. Dunn-Emke, et al. "Intensive Lifestyle Changes May Affect the Progression of Prostate Cancer." *Journal of Urology* 174.3 (September 2005): 1065–1069; discussion 1069–1070.

4. Ornish, D., M.J. Magbanua, G. Weidner, V. Weinberg, C. Kemp, C. Green, M.D. Mattie, et al. "Changes in Prostate Gene Expression in Men Undergoing an Intensive Nutrition and

Lifestyle Intervention." *Proceedings of the National Academy of Sciences USA* 105.24 (June 17, 2008): 8369–8374. (Epub June 16, 2008.)

Defining Health and Wellness

1. Prochaska, J.O., and C.C. DiClemente. "The Transtheoretical Approach." In *Handbook of Psychotherapy Integration, 2nd Ed.*, edited by J.C. Norcross and M.R. Goldfried, pp. 147–171. New York: Oxford University Press, 2005.

Step 1

1. Kabat-Zinn, Jon. *Full Catastrophe Living: Using the Wisdom of Your Body and Mind to Face Stress, Pain, and Illness.* New York: Bantam Dell, 1990.
2. Levine, Stephen. *A Year to Live: How to Live This Year as If It Were Your Last.* New York: Bell Tower, 1997.

Step 2

1. Riso, Don Richard, and Russ Hudson. *Understanding the Enneagram: The Practical Guide to Personality Types.* New York and Boston: Houghton Mifflin, 2000.
2. Riso, Don Richard, and Russ Hudson. *The Wisdom of the Enneagram: The Complete Guide to Psychological and Spiritual Growth for the Nine Personality Types.* New York: Bantam Books, 1999.

Step 3

1. Wilber, Ken. *A Brief History of Everything.* Boston, Mass.: Shambala Publications, 1996.
2. Hanh, Thich Nhat. *Peace Is Every Step.* New York: Bantam Books, 1991.

Step 4

1. "EWG's 2012 Shopper's Guide to Pesticides in Produce: USDA Dirty Dozen Plus and Clean 15." EWG.com. *www.ewg.org/food-news/summary/* (accessed June 2012).

2. Campbell, T. Colin, Thomas M. Campbell II, Howard Lyman, and John Robbins. *The China Study: The Most Comprehensive Study of Nutrition Ever Conducted and the Startling Implications for Diet, Weight Loss, and Long Term Health.* Dallas, TX.: BenBella Books, 2006.

Step 6

1. Holmes T.H, and R.H. Rahe. "The Social Readjustment Rating Scale." *Journal of Psychosomatic Research* 11.2 (1967): 213–218. Reprinted with permission from Elsevier.

Step 7

1. "Americans' Spiritual Searches Turn Inward." Gallup.com, February 11, 2003. *www.gallup.com/poll/7759/americans-spiritual-searches-turn-inward.aspx* (accessed June 2012).

2. Rohr, Richard. *Adam's Return: The Five Promises of Male Initiation.* New York: The Crossroads Publishing Company, 2004.

Resources

Checklist for group facilitators

» Consider the characteristics of group members—for example, "group of people with similar experience" or "all comers."

» Post flyer or ad for Sustainable Wellness eight-week group several weeks ahead of start date.

» Schedule a meeting place, preferably two hours per meeting, at the same time and place weekly.

» Maintain a maximum list of 12 to 14 participants for each group.

» Enlist the help of a cofacilitator, or two if possible, so there will always be a facilitator available.

» Make sure that all participants have a copy of *Sustainable Wellness* to use as a guide.

» Ask participants to provide their own journal.

» Consider having snack food or water available. Use healthy snacks and purified water.

» Begin meeting with some form of meditation or breath-focused practice from the book.

≫ Start each meeting with a reminder of the two rules for creating safe space: confidentiality and holding space for whatever comes up without trying to fix things.

≫ **First meeting:** Begin with introductions (name tags are helpful). Go around the circle clockwise, starting at the facilitator's left. All participants share their name and why they are joining the group. All participants are also asked to share one thing about themselves that they don't usually share in a social setting. After this sharing, discuss the first step as the first week's focus for practice. Go over the major review points from the chapter that corresponds to the step.

≫ Close each meeting with *Namaste*. Hold your hands in front of your chest in prayer pose and say: "I honor the place in you, where, when you are in that place in you, and I am in that place in me, there is only one of us. *Namaste*."

≫ **Week 2–7 meetings:** Begin each meeting with meditation or present-moment-awareness exercise. Then restate the two rules for safe space. Then go around the circle and allow participants to speak one at a time about their experiences with the practice for the week, or about whatever else is going on in their lives. Carefully watch for participants trying to fix another's problem, or if one participant is dominating the conversation. For example, if you spot a behavior that breaks one of the two rules, you can wonder aloud with the group at how easy it is to fall into "fixing" mode. When everyone has had a chance to talk, read the review section for the next step. If you have time, you can practice other exercises together as a group from the previous week or upcoming week. End with *Namaste*.

≫ **Week 8 meeting:** Begin the meeting with meditation or present-moment-awareness exercise. Then state the two rules for safe space. Then go around the circle and allow participants to speak one at a time about their experiences with the practice for the week, or about whatever else is going on in their lives. Close with some time for group members to speak about what the group has meant to them. You can ask them what they will be leaving behind and what they will carry forward with them. Read a poem to close and then end with *Namaste*.

≫ **After the final meeting:** Ask the participants if they would like to have further contact. Gather appropriate contact information.

>> Sign in at *www.sustainablewellnessonline.com* as a further resource to stay connected.

>> You could also consider a weekend, day, or half-day retreat during the eight-week group or afterward.

Retreat schedule example

In our retreats, in addition to having providers for cooking vegetarian food and leading massage therapy, Yoga, relaxation, and creative arts exercises, we also have an energy-medicine provider sending healing energy to all participants. All participants also fill out an application prior to the retreat with logistical information, including food and drug allergies, emergency contacts, and some questions to stimulate reflection. Before the retreat, all applications are reviewed and discussed by the facilitators and as many providers as possible. All retreat participants sign an informed participation form.

The following example is for a three-day retreat, beginning on Friday afternoon and ending on Sunday afternoon. (You can adapt this schedule for shorter or longer retreats.)

Friday	
3:00–5:00 p.m.	Arrive
5:30 p.m.	Opening session: Review logistics, rules for safe space, introductions, and sharing. Light group candle.
6:30–7:00 p.m.	Vegetarian meal, group holds silence during meal.
7:00–9:00 p.m.	Learning to stop, calm, and rest. Relaxation exercise.
9:00 p.m. until wakeup	Sleep. Holding silence after group.

Saturday	
6:30 a.m.	Wake up.
7:00–8:45 a.m.	Chair and gentle Yoga, deep relaxation.
9:00–9:30 a.m.	Breakfast, holding silence.

9:45–10:45 a.m.	Meditation practice. Introduce guided imagery (e.g., "What holds you back? What supports you? What does your ideal life look like?").
10:45 a.m.–Noon	Group split between relaxing massage by licensed therapist and spending time in nature/labyrinth.
Noon- 12:30 p.m.	Mindful, silent lunch.
12:30–1:45 p.m.	Switch groups: Massage or time in nature/labyrinth.
2:00–3:30 p.m.	Picture-drawing exercise (e.g., "What holds you back? What supports you? What does your ideal life look like?") Begin discussion of each drawing, one at a time.
3:30–3:40 p.m.	Break.
3:40–5:00 p.m.	Continue discussion of each picture, one at a time.
5:00–5:30 p.m.	Mindful meal.
5:30–8:30 p.m.	Group exercise: Forgiveness letter. Share letter as group. Outdoor fire or watch the sunset.
8:30 p.m.–Sleep	Hold silence.

Sunday	
6:30 a.m.	Wake up.
7:00–8:45 a.m.	Gentle Yoga with laughing meditation and deep relaxation.
9:00–9:30 a.m.	Breakfast. Talk about nutrition.
9:30 a.m.–Noon	Write an asking prayer, and share that prayer.
Noon–12:30 p.m.	Lunch.
12:30–2:00 p.m.	Closing ceremony. "What will I leave behind, what will I take forward?" Place group candle in protected holding area. Each participant takes home a small gift as a reminder of the retreat (we use small decorative stones).

Facilitator guidelines for retreats

Retreat preparation requires hard work, from sweeping the floors to opening the gate. It also involves the lifetime work of personal reflection and practice. As facilitators, we open the space of the heart to make room for whomever and whatever shows up.

Here we share with you some Yoga Bits that have been helpful for us and hope that you find some of them useful.

- Center yourself through a personal ritual. This might include making an asking prayer, reading a poem, sitting in meditation, or following the breath.
- Align with Spirit. "Your words, not mine."
- Similar to the tools themselves, facilitators are a neutral presence. Remember: It's not about you.
- Release attachment to any particular tool or exercise.
- None of us is a perfect vessel. Take time to review your strengths and weaknesses.
- Revisit the places where you tend to get stuck. Soften and let go of self-criticism.
- Honor other facilitators. Keep an open and respectful dialogue.
- Observe things as they unfold. The energy of a retreat ebbs and flows just like the breath.
- Focus on the present moment. Stay close to "home"; don't get lost.
- Remember: Everyone and everything has a unique timing.
- As much as possible, release personal worries and concerns. Step away from your own story.
- Listen like a sponge. No fixing.
- Hold the space widely and gently. Release attachment to outcome.
- Address the greatest need as it presents itself. Make necessary adjustments to activities along the way.
- Create a closing retreat ritual for yourself. Honor your feelings and experience.
- Step forward and begin again.

Sample Forgiveness Letter

Dear Margaret,

I've started to review my life as part of my health practice. I'm learning to pay attention to my own issues, feelings, and hurts without so much judgment and blame. It has helped me to clear out some dusty emotional "closets" and find more under-standing and compassion. After all these years, I'm aware that I still feel a little angry about the pool incident. So, I decided to work with it in my practice and write to you about the process. Here goes.

It was so long ago, but I still remember what it felt like when the bottom of the pool disappeared from under my feet and I slipped into the deep end. I was right in the middle and there was nothing to grab onto. You knew I couldn't swim. Why did you leave me alone? Somehow, I managed to kick my way to the edge of the pool and climb out. I saw you standing inside the house talking to someone at the party and having a good time. I felt so angry and embarrassed.

I realize that I've been carrying these feelings around with me all these years. Why? Why hang on to them any longer? It's time to let go—I want to let go. The love I feel for you is stronger than this childhood hurt. And I wonder how things were for you back then. It must have been hard for you to have me around all the time. You worked a lot and never really went out much. Maybe it was a special party and the only way you could go was to take me with you. I could be stubborn. Did you tell me to stay out of the pool and I got in anyway?

There are so many things that I love about you. Even when I was a kid you respected my opinions and said I could disagree as long as I was reasonable and polite. You were always there for the big things—and there were some pretty big things... It's funny, I still don't swim very well. But that's my fault, not yours. One thing I know for sure is that I'm strong enough to kick my way out of a bad situation. I learned that from you, Margaret. You're the strongest person I've ever known.

I forgive you for what happened and I'm grateful that you're part of my life. I've decided not to send this letter, but feel so much better having written it. It's almost like there's a little more space in my heart. And I'm thinking, I might just learn to swim.

Love,

Heather

Further Reading

The following are some books and resources that have inspired us.

Peace Is Every Step, Thich Nhat Hanh

Living with Uncertainty, Pema Chodron

Healing Words, Larry Dossey

Integral Spirituality, Ken Wilber

Prayers for Healing: 365 Blessings, Poems and Meditations from Around the World, Maggie Oman Shannon

One Minute Wisdom, Anthony de Mello, SJ

Adam's Return: The Five Promises of Male Initiation, Richard Rohr

Love, Medicine and Miracles, Dr. Bernie Siegel

Prescriptions for Living, Dr. Bernie Siegel

Yoga and You: Energizing and Relaxing Yoga for New and Experienced Students, Esther Myers

A Year to Live, Stephen Levine

Healthy Aging, Dr. Andrew Weil

Touch, Caring and Cancer (DVD), William Collinge

The Omnivore's Dilemma: A Natural History of Four Meals, Michael Pollan

The China Study: The Most Comprehensive Study of Nutrition Ever Conducted and the Startling Implications for Diet, Weight Loss, and Long-Term Health, T. Colin Campbell, and Thomas M. Campbell II

Index

About the Authors

Matt Mumber, MD, is a practicing, board-certified radiation oncologist with the Harbin Clinic in Rome, Georgia. He received his undergraduate and medical degrees from the University of Virginia and completed his radiation oncology residency at the Bowman Gray School of Medicine. He graduated from the 2002 Associate Fellowship Program in Integrative Medicine at the University of Arizona.

Matt serves as the medical advisor of local and regional cancer initiatives through the Georgia Cancer Coalition, and is the immediate past-president of the Georgia Society of Clinical Oncology. He founded Cancer Navigators Inc., a 501c3 corporation that provides nursing, education, and service navigation for those touched by cancer, in 2002. He continues to facilitate residential retreats for cancer patients and physicians.

Matt edited *Integrative Oncology: Principles and Practice*, published by Taylor & Francis in 2006. He is the co-director of the MD Ambassador Program at the Harbin Clinic and co-director of the Harbin Integrative Oncology Program. He received the Hamilton Jordan Founders Award in 2007 for involvement in state-wide oncology activities and was named a Health Care Hero by *Georgia Trend* magazine in 2008. He is a member of the editorial board for the *Journal of Oncology Practice* and is a past member of the Clinical Practice Committee for the American Society of Clinical Oncology. His research is focused on integrative oncology and is supported through grants as a Georgia Cancer Coalition Distinguished Scholar.

Matt and Laura enjoy raising their three children, J.T., Samson, and Marcus.

Heather Reed has been teaching Yoga in various settings since 1996. She expresses an integrative, adaptive approach and specializes in using Yoga and meditation techniques for people living with cancer, post-polio syndrome, and other chronic illnesses.

Heather received an Experienced Teacher Certification from Esther Myers Yoga Teacher Training Program and has had extensive training with senior staff of the Commonweal Cancer Help program and Dr. Dean Ornish's Program for Reversing Heart Disease. She developed Yoga classes for cancer patients at The Wellness Community in Atlanta, Georgia, where she taught from 1997 to 2004. In addition, Heather was a Yoga teacher and residential retreat facilitator for Many Streams Healing Systems, Inc., in Rome, Georgia, from 2002 to 2007. Since 2008, she has been Yoga teacher and cofacilitator for the Residential Retreat Program for Cancer Navigators of Rome, Georgia. Heather also teaches privately in Austin, Texas, where she lives with her husband and son.